PREPPER'S
SURVIVAL
MEDICINE
HANDBOOK

A Lifesaving Collection
of Emergency Procedures
from U.S. Army Field Manuals

Scott Fina___

Published in the U.S. by
ULYSSES PRESS
P.O. Box 3440
Berkeley, CA 94703
www.ulyssespress.com

ISBN: 978-1-61243-565-7
Library of Congress Control Number 2015952137

Printed in the United States

10 9 8 7 6 5 4 3 2 1

Acquisitions Editor: Casie Vogel
Managing Editor: Claire Chun
Project Editor: Caety Klingman
Editor: Lauren Harrison
Proofreader: Bill Cassel
Index: Sayre Van Young
Front cover and interior design: what!design @ whatweb.com
Layout: Jake Flaherty
Cover artwork: bloody hand © Malota/shutterstock.com, injured woman © Greg Epperson/ shutterstock.com, house/truck damage © Chad Purser/istockphoto, fire © James Brey/ istockphoto
Interior artwork: from shutterstock.com page 102 sea urchin © photossee, page 153 yucca © OK-SANA, page 184 mountain laurel © Morphart Creation, page 197 catnip © Morphart Creation

NOTE TO READERS: This book has been written and published strictly for informational and educational purposes only. It is not intended to serve as medical advice or to be any form of medical treatment. You should always consult your physician before altering or changing any aspect of your medical treatment and/or undertaking a diet regimen. Do not stop or change any prescription medications without the guidance and advice of your physician. Any use of the information in this book is made on the reader's good judgment after consulting with his or her physician and is the reader's sole responsibility. This book is not intended to diagnose or treat any medical condition and is not a substitute for a physician.

This book is independently authored and published and no sponsorship or endorsement of this book by, and no affiliation with, any trademarked brands or other products mentioned within is claimed or suggested. All trademarks that appear in this book belong to their respective owners and are used here for informational purposes only. The authors and publishers encourage readers to patronize the quality brands mentioned in this book.

*This book is dedicated to all of the men and woman who have served,
are currently serving, and will serve in the United States armed forces—
particularly my grandfather Herman Weissenborn.
You have my utmost respect and gratitude.*

CONTENTS

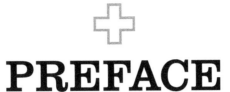

PREFACE

The calls for service that I respond to on the fire truck are met by highly trained and equipped men and women. We show up with seemingly countless hours of medical training, many years of experience, and a full complement of the latest medical equipment. Patients receive the best possible care from some of the finest people I know. Sometimes, though, a situation will arise that overwhelms our system. A weather event—a tornado, a major snowstorm, or a severe thunderstorm—will strike, and the calls for help outnumber the available resources. It's unfortunate, but those situations happen, and municipalities do the best they can with what they have.

It is in those moments that the citizens whose tax money pays for the protection of paramedics, police officers, and firefighters are forced to fend for themselves. I've seen it many times. As emergency responders establish a grip on the situation and are finally able to arrive on the scene, family, neighbors, and bystanders have rendered aid and are often simply waiting on the emergency crews to take over and transport the wounded to the hospital. They use past experience, intuition, and training to care for each other in the worst of circumstances.

Another scenario I've experienced is when injuries occur away from civilization. Someone is hiking, camping, boating, or enjoying a variety of other outdoor endeavors that put them beyond the reach of conventional communication, and suddenly they need help. The injured have no way of relaying their need for assistance. That is when first aid must be given and procedures performed because there is no one else who can help. You must then rely on the equipment and skills you have available.

The United States military has been training men and women for hundreds of years in the skills needed for survival. It places its personnel in some of the most unforgiving climates and in perilous conditions in order to carry out missions, and it is in those circumstances that they are forced to care for themselves and each other. The techniques and procedures used by our military are basic lifesaving skills that can be used by the general public in a variety of situations.

This book explains some fundamental procedures that can be used in any medical scenario. The techniques detailed in these pages can be used at the family picnic, deep in the wilderness, or in the aftermath of a natural or man-made disaster. Any time there is someone in need who can't help themselves, you have the opportunity to make a difference. It is common for survivors, or those wishing to help, to feel helpless due to lack of skills, training, and supplies. But by learning the skills covered in this book, you'll be better prepared both psychologically and physically to help out when help is needed most.

I hope you'll use this book as a resource and gather as much information as you can, and that you keep it handy as a reference to guide you through a medical emergency. Most of all, my wish is that you use this book as a springboard to seek out further medical knowledge and experience. I always say that *how you prepare is how you will respond*. Make sure you're prepared to care for those who mean the most to you at a time when they may need you the most.

However, this book is not intended to take the place of any formal medical training. It is based on information gathered from U.S. military manuals and field guides. I have also added advice from my own training and experience as a firefighter. If you have the ability to call for paramedic help or take the injured person to a doctor or hospital, you should do so. Only turn to the advice in this book when the disaster situation is such that you have no other option.

✛
INTRODUCTION

For centuries soldiers have been sent to battlefields, and over the course of their missions, there was one inevitability: There would be casualties. U.S. military personnel are trained in nearly every conceivable area of combat and survival. They are prepared and equipped to be self-reliant in a variety of situations and climates. A constant state of readiness is an absolute must because they could be called into action at any time and, more often than not, they are called to areas and conditions where they are unsupported. It is never a question of *if*—it is a matter of *when*.

One area where they must be extremely proficient is that of first aid. Soldiers do dangerous work in dangerous conditions, and one inherent consequence of that is the likelihood of injury. They must know how to respond, at a moment's notice, to any possible medical emergency. While some are trained and certified doctors and nurses, many are just like you. They have no formal medical background or education. They have other specialties that they are responsible for knowing, yet when something goes wrong, they want and are expected to be able to help their fellow soldiers or civilians. Where they go, there is no option to call an ambulance or have a doctor or other medical professional there to render care. They must be able to treat each other, and often themselves, in less than ideal conditions and with minimal equipment.

The conditions in which military personnel are forced to perform first aid are not dissimilar to what civilians frequently experience in the hours following a disaster. Disasters, both natural and man-made, strike all too often and leave a path of people reeling in their wake trying to care for themselves and each other. Untrained citizens do what they can with what they have available.

It is primal instinct, self-preservation, that drives us to try to heal ourselves when we're injured and there is no one else to help. It's also human nature to reach out to others when they can't help themselves. Despite how dark and bleak society can seem at times, one thing that disasters have taught us is that we, human beings, will help one another. Yes, there are those who will take advantage and capitalize on tragedy, but the vast majority of people can be seen in the wilderness or atop piles of debris, among the broken pieces of what once was their world, doing whatever they can to help each other. They don't do it for notoriety; they do it because there is someone who needs help and there may be no one else around.

Whether you're alone in a remote area, away from the comfortable reach of civil services such as an ambulance, police, or fire department, or a catastrophic event has occurred and the system becomes overwhelmed, there are situations in which you may realistically find that the only help available is yourself. Medical emergencies are unpredictable and can vary from superficial to deadly. Your best chance of being able to render aid is to know basic, yet lifesaving procedures that can greatly affect the well-being of a sick or injured person.

When that time comes, you will naturally revert to any previous experience or training you have. Regardless of what you bring to the table, whether it's years of experience in emergency medicine, or little experience and simply this book, one thing you should always maintain is a sense of control and calm. The victim will likely be anxious and scared. Part of your job as a caregiver is to display a calm demeanor that will reap psychological and potentially medical benefits for your patient or patients. One of the easiest things to do is to let anxiety dictate your thoughts and actions, but, as Rudyard Kipling writes, "If you can keep your head when all about you are losing theirs," you will enjoy a far greater likelihood of positive outcomes.

In my 15 years of service as a military medic, I have had only a few occasions to interact with the patients I have treated after they left my care. Not a single one mentioned any specific treatment or technique that I used to manage their injuries, but all of them commented something about how having a calm person at their side during crisis eased and comforted them. I believe that in addition to knowing the essentials of first aid, it is imperative to make a plan and mentally rehearse the first step of responding to an emergency of any kind: staying calm and conveying confidence to those who need your assistance. It's not likely that anyone will remember the exact way that you stopped their bleeding, splinted their injury, or treated their shock, but they almost certainly will remember your tone and non-anxious presence during their most difficult moments. This can make all the difference to their long-term recovery, both physical and mental.

Angela Caruso-Yahne,
Aeromedical Technician,
United States Air Force

I write this book not as an experienced military veteran, but as a career firefighter who has spent two decades responding to medical calls and acknowledges the stellar training and proven procedures that the United States military provides. I have many coworkers, friends, and family members who have served or are currently serving in our armed forces in various capacities. It is in the stories they've shared and the conversations we've had that the idea for this book was born. The men and women who dedicate their lives to the service and protection of our nation all too often must utilize these medical aid procedures.

Unfortunately, the competencies detailed in this book are not just words on a page. They are methods that, if used correctly and at the right time, could be the difference between life and death. More commonly, though, they will be used to effectively treat a common injury for someone who is in need. These are skills taught to our service members that are practical, efficient, and proven, and could and should be used by civilians—civilians who find themselves in need of expedient medical aid by a trained and equipped professional medical crew when that is not an option.

The intent of this book is not to make you a medical expert. This book offers basic procedures taken from U.S. military manuals, as well as my years of experience running thousands of medical calls on the big red fire truck. My goal for you, the reader, is to absorb the content of this book, practice the procedures found here, ask questions and seek answers, and use this as both a reference and a launching point for your medical training. This book will serve its purpose after you have read it, sitting on your shelf where you can reach it if needed or in the backpack or first aid kit that you take with you to respond to an emergency. *Prepper's Survival Medicine Handbook* will achieve its maximum potential if you practice and become proficient in the skills contained here and are prepared to help even a single person who could not otherwise help themselves. Pursue training classes, educational opportunities, and circumstances to practice and hone your patient assessment and treatment skills.

Note: With the full respect and acknowledgment that "soldier" often refers to a member of the Army, while other branches use "troop," "sailor," "marine," etc., this book will commonly make references to "soldiers" as a general term for all members of our armed forces. I humbly thank each and every one of you for your service.

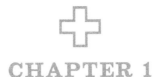

CHAPTER 1

BASIC PROCEDURES

BEING READY VERSUS BEING PREPARED

It's semantics, really—"ready" versus "prepared." One could argue they're the same thing. In fact, if you look one up in a thesaurus, you'll find the other listed as a synonym, and throughout this book they will be used synonymously. However, certain distinctions have been made when it comes to disaster preparation.

Being prepared implies physical readiness. It means you have obtained the supplies and skills needed to respond to an event that would render you and your family without the ability to receive emergency help. You have gathered the right things, stored the appropriate supplies, read the books, and practiced the survival techniques that you'll need when the time arises. The work has been done in advance.

Being ready, on the other hand, is having the mental and emotional capacity not only to endure a catastrophic event, but also to perform under the direst of circumstances. When your everyday life is disrupted and you are forced to be self-reliant, it can be a frightening experience. Regardless of how *prepared* you are, it doesn't necessarily mean you are *ready* to undertake the responsibility of ensuring safety, food, water, and shelter for you and your family. From experience I can tell you that it is one thing to perform first aid on someone, but another thing entirely to be in a situation where you have to render care to yourself or a loved one. Practically speaking, first aid is the same, regardless of the patient. The same procedures are performed, the same precautions are taken. But the reality is that there is a heightened sense of urgency, and even stress, when you're taking care of someone you know. This can become especially problematic for those who already have anxiety issues or have suffered post-traumatic stress.

So the question is, how does one ensure both preparation and readiness? The answer is that it's completely up to you. My comfort level for preparation is going to differ from yours, just as yours will differ from the next person's. But there are some basic supplies, reference materials, and skills that should be considered a minimum in survival medicine, and those will be discussed throughout this book. Personal readiness? That begins with identifying what disasters are most common for your area. Do you live along the Gulf Coast where hurricanes are a perennial threat? Is your city in the Midwest under continual tornado watches and warnings every spring? Is there the potential for wildfires, mudslides, industrial accidents, or even civil unrest or terrorist attacks near you? Identifying this can help you begin to wrap your mind around what could potentially be expected of you.

The whole process of looking ahead and planning for a worst-case scenario can be overwhelming and create more than its fair share of anxiety. This book will discuss a vast number of medical scenarios that will help to prepare you. The U.S. military's *Medical Platoon Leaders' Handbook* outlines medical divisions within the military and describes them as largely self-sustaining and capable of independent operations. This book will apply the same philosophy, outlining different scenarios that will help you quickly and easily access the right information for the right circumstance. With the information contained here, you should be able to operate independently until emergency responders can arrive and take over the patient care that you started.

GOOD HEALTH AND PHYSICAL FITNESS

What comes to mind when you think about readying yourself for disaster? Food? Water? Shelter? First aid? Of course. These are all critically important and should not be discounted. But one of the most often overlooked areas is that of personal health. There are many reasons why good health and physical fitness should be top priorities, not only in your disaster preparation, but in life in general. According to the President's Council on Fitness, Sports, and Nutrition, one-third of Americans are obese. With obesity comes serious health risks such as high blood pressure, diabetes, heart disease, and cancer. You'll be doing yourself a great disservice if you take measures to ensure your disaster readiness but neglect your own physical fitness.

Be honest with yourself about your level of fitness. The *US Army Survival Manual* states, "Prepare yourself to cope with the rigors of survival." When you're in a disaster situation, consider the types of activities you may be forced to perform: escaping dangerous situations, hiking long distances, climbing over rubble, carrying and dragging victims, digging, hoisting, lifting heavy loads, clearing away debris, and numerous other labor-intensive activities. Disasters are physically demanding, and to be ready, you should be in good health and physically fit.

A good physical fitness routine combines a healthy diet, cardiovascular fitness, and weight training. To neglect any one of the three areas could lead to dire consequences, particularly in a crisis situation. Eating a balanced diet inclusive of protein, fruits, and vegetables will keep your energy up and afford you a baseline level of good health.

The benefits of cardiovascular fitness go far beyond being "in shape." Often people think of cardiovascular exercise as a way to burn off excess calories and lose weight, but there are many more reasons to maintain a good level of cardio. You've no doubt heard that your heart is a muscle and must be exercised. Cardiovascular exercises, such as walking, jogging, and swimming, increase your heart rate and strengthen the cardiac muscle. Other benefits include increased metabolism and an improved hormonal profile, which means reduced symptoms of fatigue and depression.

Finally, weight training should be included in your fitness regimen. That doesn't mean you need to be a bodybuilder, unless that is a specific goal of yours. It simply means that strength is needed in everyday life, but particularly during a crisis. Strength training protects bone health and muscle mass, boosts energy levels, and aids in better body mechanics, including posture, flexibility, and balance.

SURVIVAL

The *US Army Survival Manual* uses the acronym SURVIVAL to guide your actions. While their explanation is broader, here we'll focus on how this acronym pertains specifically to emergency medicine.

S: Size up the situation. (surroundings, physical condition, equipment)

U: Use all of your senses.

R: Remember where you are.

V: Vanquish fear and panic.

I: Improvise.

V: Value living.

A: Act like the natives.

L: Live by your wits, but for now, learn basic skills.

SIZE UP THE SITUATION

"Size-up" is a term used by the military and emergency responders to refer to the process of quickly evaluating a situation. Whatever the circumstances, before you decide on a course of action, you need to quickly, and as accurately as possible, determine three things: 1. What has happened to cause this? 2. What is happening now? 3. What is going to happen? By doing this you use a combination of your senses and your experience to develop a strategy for the most appropriate and safest response.

Determining cause is extremely important. One of the most important lessons in rendering aid to someone is to not become part of the problem. You should take all measures to keep yourself, and anyone else rendering aid, as safe as possible. One of the first ways to do that is to ensure you aren't putting yourself directly in harm's way by helping. For example, if the cause of this medical emergency is weather related, there are ways to find out if the event is over or if it is going to continue. If there has been an explosion or a hazardous materials leak, you may not have any idea if it's safe to enter the area and begin treatment. In fact, you stand a better chance than not of turning rescuers into victims by sending them in to the unknown. By determining what caused the medical emergency, you can better decide the best way to offer aid. Sometimes there is no way to accurately determine what has happened and if it is completely safe for rescuers to approach the scene, but by using your senses and intuition, you should make the best determination for the greater good.

The second part of your size-up is evaluating the scene as it is right now. As a firefighter, I'm often called to medical scenes where we arrive and I have to make a quick assessment of what we're dealing with. Once it has been determined (as much as possible) that it is safe to send rescue workers in, you have to assess what is happening now. How many victims are there? What are the primary medical issues? Is it a respiratory issue, burns, bleeding, etc.? Do you have the right amount of people and supplies to handle the situation? Sometimes, *more* isn't an option, and your only choice is to do the best you can with what you have available.

And finally, you should predict what is about to happen. Is the situation going to get worse or better? If the answer is "worse," what are your options? Can you somehow stop the cause of what has happened? Can you relocate victims? Are you going to need more rescuers, medical supplies, or vehicles to transport patients? Even dating back to the Vietnam war era, according to *The Aidman's Medical Guide*, military medical operations were set up where you are "readily accessible to expected patients and where your men know they can find you."

Size-up is the first thing you will do as you approach a disaster scene, but it doesn't end there. It is an ongoing process that should be done over and over again throughout the incident. Consistent reevaluation will keep you and your fellow rescuers aware of your surroundings and situation. But size-up isn't just for the overall incident. It's done when treating patients as well. What has happened to the person? What is the resulting illness or injury? What can you do about it? If that doesn't work, what's your plan B? Then, constantly reevaluate to determine if what you're doing is having the desired outcome for overall patient care.

USE ALL OF YOUR SENSES

A good size-up will draw from all of your senses—all *six* of them, the sixth one being your instinct. U.S. military survival guides caution against moving just for the sake of taking action. Acting in haste can have negative repercussions and dangerous consequences for both you and your patients. Most of us naturally want to spring into action when we see someone in need. But there are certain levels of safety and protection that must be utilized that we will cover in detail later in this chapter.

Sight: What do you see? What is the extent of the illness or injury? Are there trapped victims? Are you in a safe area or should you relocate?

Sound: Is anyone yelling for help? Can you hear gas leaking or water running? Do you hear approaching sirens? What are your patients telling you?

Smell: Do you smell smoke, natural gas, or any other suspicious odors?

Touch: Is your patient hot to the touch? Cold to the touch? Does something feel abnormal? Broken?

Taste: Believe it or not, there are taste receptors located in the smooth muscle of your trachea and bronchi. If you have an odd taste in your mouth with no reasonable explanation, that may be a warning that you've inhaled an irritant of some kind and should evaluate the possible hazard and consider evacuating to a safer location.

Instinct: Trust it. Even if there is no obvious evidence suggesting you take or avoid a particular course of action, your instinct could quite possibly be a subconscious recognition of something that you couldn't otherwise identify.

REMEMBER WHERE YOU ARE

As elementary as it sounds, know where you are. What is your location in the city, area, or building? That specific information will be critical when coordinating rescue efforts or working with emergency responders who are trying to reach you. If it's a large-scale incident, you should be able to identify your location by the specific address or nearest intersection (for example, you could let emergency responders know you have eight patients near the intersection of Third and Main Streets). If the event occurs in your office building, it would be beneficial to determine, for example, that you are on the second floor in the north stairwell. Large-scale incidents will require you to know that information so you are able to specify an area to gather patients and coordinate their removal for transport.

You'll also want to know where you are in proximity to potential hazards. The general rule for rendering aid is to try to pick a location that is uphill and upwind from harm. This will reduce the risk of inadvertently conducting your operations in the path of danger. But keep in mind changing wind conditions. It's common for wind to shift direction with little warning, which can put you and any patients receiving care in the path of anything from foul odors to harmful gases. Be aware of your location.

VANQUISH FEAR AND PANIC

Cus D'Amato, trainer for former heavyweight boxing champion Mike Tyson, once said, "Fear is like fire. It can cook for you. It can heat your house. Or it can burn you down." Unless they are controlled, your worst enemies during a crisis can be fear and panic. No one is immune to fear, but the ability to control it can be the difference between success and failure. The amount of stress placed on disaster survivors can be intense and can have adverse effects on their mental health, physical health, and ability to make good decisions. Stress causes the release of cortisol, adrenaline, and other hormones that interfere with your brain's ability to accurately perceive your surroundings and to make decisions. Under stress it is common for your field of vision to narrow and to focus on one specific thing, which can leave you vulnerable in a dangerous environment.

By taking a moment, if the situation allows, to gather yourself and take a breath before acting, you'll tend to act more on logic than emotion. Those decisions are made through what Laurence Gonzales, in his book *Deep Survival: Who Lives, Who Dies, and Why*, calls "emotional bookmarks." He says, "The emotional system reacts to circumstances, finds bookmarks that flag similar experiences in your past and your response to them, and allows you to recall the feelings, good or bad, of the outcome of your actions." The best way to vanquish fear and panic is to utilize the self-confidence that comes with preparation and training.

IMPROVISE

If you're the type of person who is so structured that the thought of improvising creates an increased heart rate and sweaty palms, you may find yourself dangerously out of your comfort zone during a crisis. The ability to improvise is not only recommended, but an absolute necessity. No matter how thorough your preparations and training, fate will find a way to overwhelm you or throw you a curveball, and you must be able to make do. You may not have at your disposal sterile gauze to wrap a laceration, but you can find a clean cloth or even use superglue to close a wound.

VALUE LIVING

In any type of disaster response there are incident priorities that are the same for emergency responders, military, and civilians alike. Regardless of your background or how you came to be there, your priorities always begin with life safety. Life safety is the number one priority in any incident (followed by incident stabilization and property conservation). Rescuer safety should be given equal or even higher consideration than that of the victims. That may be a bitter pill to swallow, but in a mass-casualty incident, victims are going to outnumber rescuers. It is imperative that rescuers are kept as safe as possible in order to do the greatest amount of good for the greatest number of people. That is a recurring theme in this book: *Do the greatest amount of good for the greatest number of people.* If you are rendering aid, you need to value your life as much as those you are trying to help. The Federal Aviation Administration (FAA) requires flight attendants to remind you of this before the takeoff of every flight: If there is a drop in cabin pressure, oxygen masks will drop from the compartment above you, and you should place your mask over your mouth and nose before helping others. You don't become a hero by becoming a victim.

ACT LIKE THE NATIVES

The *US Army Survival Manual* says to act like the natives as a survival tactic in deployed combat situations. For our purposes, we'll take a slightly different approach while applying the idea's core principle: adaptation to your environment. The manual says that you should utilize the natives to find food, water, and shelter, and to observe their actions in order to fit in and avoid capture. It's a lesson in adaptation. In emergency medicine, adapting to your environment is an absolute necessity. Makeshift treatment areas are thrown up in far less than ideal locations. Survivors adapt to their environment and make do with what is available. The "natives" or, more likely, the locals, the occupants, or anyone else with knowledge of the building or area, can be a great asset as you begin to render aid to victims.

LIVE BY YOUR WITS, BUT FOR NOW, LEARN BASIC SKILLS

The time to learn the basics is before an event occurs. Begin now. There are vast amounts of literature available, and more classes than you are probably aware of right in your area. Local colleges, parks and recreation commissions, the Red Cross, the Salvation Army, fire departments, and a variety of other groups and organizations offer classes on a regular basis that are low cost or even free of charge. Take advantage of as many of those opportunities as you can. You'll not only learn and reinforce medical skills, but you'll also have the opportunity to network with people in your area.

It's one thing to read about skills, but it's another thing entirely to practice them. Many medical scenarios can be difficult to "practice," such as the recognition of shock or treating low blood sugar, but there are other skills where practice can create a level of proficiency that will reduce stress during a time of crisis. If you are able to control bleeding, position an airway, or splint a fracture confidently, you will experience less anxiety and be better prepared to aid those around you when you are called upon to help.

SCENE SAFETY

Imagine a crisis situation in which you have to render aid. What are you going to do about it? What do you mean you don't know? Why not? Because you don't know what it is you're getting into? That's a good point. You're right. You need one thing: information. My point is that emergency responders every day respond to crisis situations and arrive with very limited information. As an officer with the fire department, on *every* emergency scene, I do a quick size-up and determine scene safety by rapidly taking in and processing information. As I mentioned before, I'm using my senses. I'm using what bystanders tell me. I'm looking for anything that could pose a threat to those preparing to provide aid. I'm also looking for anything that could cause further harm to victims.

There are both big and small issues that you should look for, such as obvious hazardous material leaks, building collapse, fire, dangerous animals, traffic, downed power lines, or a person or people wishing to do harm. If one of those, or anything else you deem potentially harmful, is present, you will want to exercise extreme caution before approaching the scene.

Some of these things are obvious hazards, and we have limited ability to control them. One of the first steps in determining whether a scene is safe is acknowledging that you are dealing with the unpredictable. The most predictable element of the scene is you. You control where you go, what you do, where you walk, and how you operate. Scene safety will require constant evaluation. You must be aware and remain aware of the things around you that can hurt or kill you.

PERSONAL PROTECTIVE EQUIPMENT

The use of personal protective equipment (PPE) cannot be stressed enough. Simply put, PPE consists of the items you wear to keep yourself as safe as possible in an unsafe environment. You use PPE every day and don't even realize it. Do you use sunscreen in the summer? PPE. Do you wear your seat belt? PPE. Do you wear a hat and gloves in the winter? PPE. Do you use an oven mitt to remove a hot pan from the oven? PPE. You see where I'm going with this. We utilize personal protective equipment in our daily lives. In a disaster situation, we take things one step further. You will be dealing with potentially harsh weather conditions, uneven terrain, jagged metal, and other safety hazards. Gloves, safety glasses, weather-appropriate clothing, and things of that nature are all common items that you should keep around.

PPE also encompasses body substance isolation (BSI) gear. BSI means you are taking measures to reduce the chance of transmitting pathogens (bacteria, viruses, or other microorganisms that can cause disease). That's why surgeons wear surgical masks, gowns, eye protection, and gloves. For the record, BSI *is* personal protective equipment, but I'll address it specifically because of its relevance when talking about anything medical. The U.S. Air Force states in its *Infection Prevention and Control Program* publication that, "Personnel will wear PPE

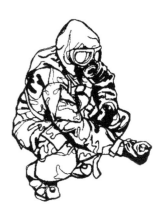

Example of PPE

(e.g., gloves, gowns, goggles, masks) appropriate for the task to form a personal barrier of protection for associated exposure risk per standard precaution." It goes on to add that: "Personnel will wear PPE appropriate for the task to form a barrier of protection against exposure of blood, other body fluids, infections and chemical agents from contamination of clinical attire, undergarments, skin, eyes, mouth, or other mucous membranes under normal conditions of use and for the duration of time which the PPE will be used."

Any type of first aid training begins with two things: scene safety and BSI. Once you have determined the scene to be safe, or safe enough to render aid, your next step is to ensure you have BSI in place. Just like a surgeon, practicing good BSI means blocking any possible route for an exchange of fluid. This means from you to the victim as well as from the victim to you.

Skin: Skin is the largest organ in your body and provides multiple layers of protection. All in all, human skin does an exceptional job of keeping unwanted bacteria and viruses out of our bodies. However, if there is a break in the skin, be it a cut or scrape or even a tiny imperfection that compromises the full thickness of protection that skin provides, bad things can find their way into your bloodstream. Protect the skin by being completely covered with clothing that offers at least some measure of barrier protection.

Eyes: Eyes must be protected for multiple reasons, but when thinking about BSI, you must know that the eyes provide a direct route into your body and should be protected at all times. When providing any first aid, never neglect eye protection. Safety glasses or a surgical mask with an eye shield should be worn any time you're providing patient care.

Mouth and nose: Similar to the eyes, the mouth and nose do not offer much protection for your bloodstream and should be provided the same level of protection. The large number of mucous membranes in these areas offer a dangerously easy route for the transmission of blood-borne pathogens. The most common method of providing barrier protection for the mouth and nose is a surgical mask. They are inexpensive and can be found in many prepackaged first aid kits.

Hands: The hands are one of the most common areas for contamination. Especially in the period immediately following a disaster, it's a perfect storm: large number of victims, limited number of rescuers, PPE not readily available. When you render aid to someone, whether they are bleeding or not, you should *always* use gloves. In recent years, the medical industry has moved away from using latex gloves due to the large number of latex allergies and more often uses nitrile gloves.

Other, more general personal protective equipment could include any or all of the following:

+ Sturdy shoes

+ Weather-appropriate clothing

+ Leather gloves

+ Hard hat

+ Sunscreen

+ Safety glasses

+ Hearing protection

+ Respirator

+ Reflective vest

+ Any other personal protective equipment needed for your specific situation

MEDICAL SIZE-UP

Medical size-up utilizes the same principles that were previously discussed with scene size-up in that you're using your experience, intuition, and senses to determine a course of action. With medical size-up, though, you're focusing specifically on patient care. The first two steps of a good medical size-up are, of course, scene safety and PPE. Once you've checked those off your list, you'll begin with the big picture and then narrow your focus. As with other forms of size-up, it really comes down to three things: 1) What happened/what are you dealing with? 2) What do you want to do about it? 3) What is your backup plan? Medical scenarios are no different.

Once scene safety and PPE have been established, you'll need to determine the number of patients. This is not a time for treatment. It's not even a time to begin prioritizing patients by severity of their injuries. This is a very quick overview of the situation at hand. Determining the number of victims is very important, but can be deceiving. Even a few patients can be overwhelming if there are significant injuries and not enough people and supplies to adequately help.

Only you will be able to evaluate if the resources you have available are adequate to satisfy the need. You may need to gather more help or render aid based on priority. If there are up to four patients, this might not be an issue, but if you're dealing with a mass-casualty incident, such as a bus crash, riot, or major weather event, the number of patients could be vast. Do the best you can to quickly verify how many people are going to require medical aid.

Next, you will consider mechanism of injury (MOI), which is a different way of saying "what caused the injury." This is important for several reasons. First and foremost, you'll need to know if the event is over. It can be difficult and dangerous to provide "battlefield medicine." Even military medics will tell you that, given the opportunity, they'll provide much better patient care once the soldier is off the battlefield and in a somewhat controlled environment. The other important factor with mechanism of injury is that by knowing what caused the issue, you can be more aware of the potential injuries. There are certain injuries that correlate with a specific MOI. With an explosion you can expect burns, concussion-related internal injuries, hearing problems, possible amputations, and so on. If there was a carbon monoxide leak into an occupied building, you can expect more respiratory issues, chest pain, vomiting, confusion, and things of that nature. By identifying the MOI, you're better prepared to treat those who are affected.

Finally, you'll need to make the determination of what additional resources you'll need. Often, following a disaster, receiving more of anything isn't an option. You must make do with what you have available. But you should still make a mental "wish list" of what is required—be it people, supplies, and transport options—to adequately treat the number of patients in your care. As options become available, you'll already have a rough idea of what you may need. At some point, preferably sooner rather than later, other people will arrive to help, and most of them will want something to do. They're there to be a part of the solution. If you've done an adequate size-up, you can immediately tell them where the greatest need is, whether it's patient care, gathering first aid supplies, or finding more people to help.

Once you're ready to begin patient care, each individual patient will receive their *own* size-up. You'll make a determination of the possible illness or injury, the severity, and the treatment options. As we progress through this book, you'll learn how to recognize and how to deal with specific medical issues. Before any treatment begins, you must figure out, to the best of your ability, what you are treating and why. Have you ever gone to the doctor and he or she immediately starts treating the injury or giving you medicine without asking you questions? No. They must first perform a size-up. What happened? How did it happen? What hurts? Does anything make the pain/condition better or worse? Does it hurt anywhere else? Has this happened before? Again, information is the key to the best possible patient care. Sometimes, if the victim is unconscious or confused, you won't have the luxury of information. You'll have to make educated guesses based on what you observe and what you know through training.

Performing a quick and thorough medical size-up will put you in the best possible place to begin making a bad situation better. It will ensure that you have considered rescuer safety and have a thought process for the best course of action. Human beings are both gifted and flawed by the power of our emotions. At our core, there is a drive for survival. When someone is in need, we want to help. Unfortunately, our emotions often overtake rational thought and cause us to focus on a specific task, meaning we may miss bigger-picture things such as safety issues. The instinctive desire to help can be dangerous if we don't consciously take a moment to size up the situation.

SIGNS AND SYMPTOMS

Signs are something that can be seen (sweating, bleeding, bruising, etc.).

Symptoms are felt (chest pain, headache, nausea, etc.).

ABCs

While life safety is the first and foremost priority in any situation, within that category there are other priorities as well. If you think about it, the body is an incredibly resilient object. Actually, it's a collection of many systems all miraculously working together in perfect harmony to keep us breathing, moving, feeling, and living. It's possible to lose limbs or certain organs and still live a long and happy life. There are some things, though, that are an absolute requirement. In an emergency situation, responders assess the patient's ABCs: airway, breathing, and circulation.

AIRWAY AND BREATHING

Your body not only requires oxygen to survive, but requires a specific amount. The air we breathe every day contains around 21 percent oxygen. The rest is made up of mostly nitrogen and a few other gases, but it is right around that 21 percent oxygen mark that allows us to live and function normally. When talking about oxygenating the body, airway and breathing are often used synonymously. Airway, more specifically, refers to the pathway of moving air and the physical occlusions that could hinder that process. Breathing is the process of getting oxygen into your lungs and bloodstream, and the ability to exhale carbon dioxide.

Your trachea, also known as your windpipe or your airway, provides a pathway for oxygen to get to your lungs. The airway can only perform its task of providing that pathway if it is clear and free of obstructions. If the tube becomes blocked, air can't move through it, reducing or completely eliminating one's ability to breathe.

According to *The Special Operation Forces Medical Handbook*, respiratory examination should include inspection of chest, percussion of chest, palpation of chest, and auscultation of lungs. This is to be done only if the casualty count is low enough that you can give your patient a thorough and focused exam. In a mass-casualty incident, simply look and listen for breathing and feel for a chest rise.

CIRCULATION

The unobstructed airway and the process of breathing are all in place in order for your body to be able to move oxygenated blood to the muscle and tissue that requires it. That oxygenated blood is pumped by the heart. Your heart is about the size of your fist and sits in the middle of your chest. Blood receives its oxygen in the lungs and then goes to the heart to be circulated around the body to the muscles, organs, and tissues that need it. If for whatever reason the heart stops pumping, it is imperative that a rescuer begin to force oxygenated blood throughout the body by way of chest compressions.

When the brain is deprived of oxygen, brain damage can begin within four minutes and become irreversible within seven minutes. To keep the brain functioning normally, an open airway is required, as well as intact breathing and the ability for the heart to circulate the oxygenated blood throughout the body. When the ABCs are not intact, immediate intervention is required.

In 2010, the American Heart Association reprioritized the ABCs to Circulation, Airway, Breathing (CAB) to put more emphasis on circulation, but the medical community still uses ABC, with airway at the top of the list. Later, we'll discuss how to check for an open airway, breathing, circulation, and options for intervention, but for now, you should know that when you perform any kind of assessment, it always begins with the ABCs.

HELPFUL RESOURCES

It is always helpful to have first aid literature, books, and field manuals handy in case you need a quick reference to give medical aid to yourself or someone else. Small books and field guides in particular fit easily into a backpack or first aid kit where they can be portable and readily available in a time of need. However, just having a good guide is usually not enough to administer proper medical care. To truly be ready for any emergency, you need a fully stocked first aid kit, proper training and certification, and as many additional resources as possible.

FIRST AID SUPPLIES

Administering first aid can be challenging, particularly if you're in an environment that's not *controlled*. An uncontrolled environment is basically anywhere that doesn't offer sterile and sanitary facilities and supplies for patient care. Whatever circumstances have led you to have to provide field treatment for yourself or others, you'll want to have the appropriate supplies, which isn't always possible.

Having a fully stocked first aid kit will offer you the best treatment options, so you should have as complete an inventory as possible. We'll discuss other possible options for the times you don't have access to your kit, but to give yourself the best possible advantage for rendering care, you should have first aid supplies that include any or all of the following:

- ❑ Field first aid guide

- ❑ PPE (such as sterile gloves, safety glasses, medical masks)

- ❑ Alcohol-based hand sanitizer (at least 60 percent alcohol)

- ❑ 4 x 4-inch gauze

- ❑ 2 x 2-inch gauze

- ❑ Roll gauze

- ❑ Medical tape (one each of paper, plaster, Micropore)

- ❑ Antibacterial ointment

- ❑ Variety-size package of adhesive bandages

- ❑ Butterfly bandages

- ❑ Superglue

- ❑ Normal saline

- ❑ Burn dressing

- ❑ Triangular bandages (with safety pins)

- ❑ Cotton swabs

- ❑ Ice packs

- ❑ Heat packs

- ❑ Trauma shears

- ❑ Tweezers

- ❑ Thermometer (with protective cover)

- ❑ Pain reliever (such as acetaminophen, ibuprofen)

- ❑ Aspirin

- ❑ Aloe vera gel

- ❑ Antihistamine (Benadryl)

- ❑ Insect bite treatment

- ❑ Antidiarrheal medication

- ❑ Antacid

- ❑ Prescription medication (such as high blood pressure medication or insulin)

- ❑ Activated charcoal

- ❑ Petroleum jelly

- ❑ Cold/flu medication

- ❑ Eye drops

- ❑ Snakebite kit

- ❑ Emergency dental kit

These items should suffice for a basic first aid kit and could be useful in treating a wide range of injuries. However, there are times when you won't have a first aid kit at hand and will be forced to rely on what you have available, which could mean utilizing some unconventional items or methods to render first aid. In a survival situation, you'll find and benefit from many items that have multiple uses.

Tampons and maxi pads: They are manufactured for one specific purpose—to absorb blood. Tampons can be used to treat a bloody nose or a puncture wound. (They can also be pulled apart to use as kindling to start a fire.) Unscented maxi pads work extremely well as a dressing used to treat any kind of bleeding injury.

Duct tape: Duct tape is one of the greatest multiuse items you can have in any disaster preparation kit. For first aid, it's used to secure dressings and splints, and it is strong enough to create a makeshift stretcher. Put a roll in your kit and you'll be amazed at the problems you can solve with duct tape.

Plastic bags: Everything from trash bags to sandwich-sized sealable bags are good to have in your supplies. I've also found that keeping first aid supplies separated by sealable plastic bags is a good way to organize

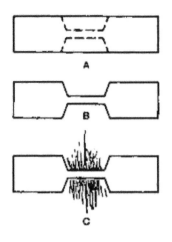

Example of a butterfly bandage

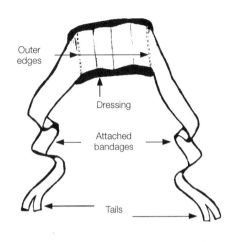

Example of a burn dressing

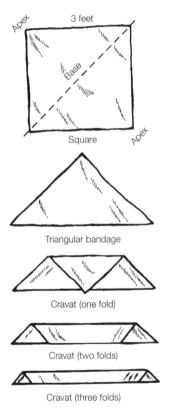

Triangular and cravat bandages

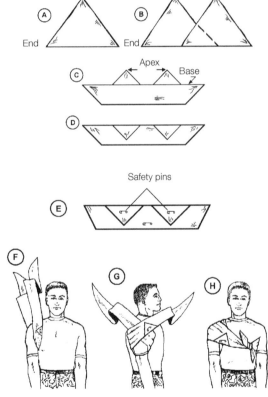

Extended cravat bandage applied to shoulder

your kit, as well as to have a few extra bags for varying uses. Bags can obviously be used for keeping items dry or for containing medical waste, or even to protect wounds or burns from infection until advanced care can be reached.

Safety pins: Some first aid kits contain safety pins, but many do not. They can be used to hold bandages or splints in place. Another use is to dig out splinters. There are more general uses as well, such as holding fabric together on a torn shirt or pants.

Tea bags: Tea leaves have anti-inflammatory and vasoconstrictive (blood vessel–narrowing) properties that can be used to slow blood loss. To receive the maximum benefit from tea bags, pour just enough boiling water on the bag to make it swell so that only a small amount of liquid is leaking from it. Once it has sufficiently cooled, you can apply it to a nosebleed, a wound, or even a tooth socket in the case of a traumatic tooth extraction. The tannin in the tea leaves will cause the blood vessels to constrict, reducing blood loss.

Vapor rub: There are several common medical uses for vapor rub, but one that you won't find on the label is to prevent distracting, foul-smelling odors from hindering your first aid efforts. Often in a disaster scenario there are awful odors of wound infection, death, and/or human waste. By putting a generous dab under your nostrils, you can better avoid succumbing to the potentially gut-wrenching odors.

Liquid bandage: This product has been sold on first aid shelves for years, but surprisingly isn't well-known beyond outdoorsy types of people. It's a small container of liquid that when dropped onto a wound dries within minutes to form a protective layer on top. It is incredibly easy to apply and provides an excellent barrier against dirt, water, and germs.

Credit card: An old credit card, debit card, library card, grocery store rewards card, or any other firm card is a good item to have handy in certain medical situations. It can be used to scrape against the skin to remove a stinger in the case of an insect sting, or it can be cut up and used to splint fingers or toes.

Frozen vegetables: In the event that you need an ice pack but don't have one readily available, you can always grab a bag of frozen vegetables out of the freezer to serve the same purpose. If possible, use a bag of peas as they mold nicely around an injured area to help reduce inflammation and swelling.

Candy: It's amazing how a piece of candy can help an injured person's spirit. This is especially true of children, although it works for adults too. A small bag of hard candies with a long shelf life is a nice bonus to add to your kit.

There are many options when selecting items to place in your first aid kid or to utilize when rendering first aid. The one simple piece of advice is to do no harm. As long as you're helping the situation, or at the very least preventing a situation from getting worse, you're doing the right thing. You should use caution when using home remedies. For example, for years it was widely thought that placing butter on a burn would help to seal it off from air and bacteria, aiding the healing process. However, putting butter or a similar substance on a burn actually hinders the release of heat, which worsens the burn.

Stick with safe, tried-and-true methods for rendering first aid. Sure, you may have to use duct tape to secure a bandage, which is something you would never see in an emergency room, but it is a safe, non-invasive procedure. In a critical situation, do what you need to in the best interest of the patient, as long as you aren't experimenting or doing anything to worsen the situation. It's always best to have medical supplies close at hand, but remember, the most useful first aid items you can have are training and experience.

FOOD SUPPLIES

Many medical issues, such as high and low blood pressure, diabetes, dehydration, and shock can be helped by ingesting food and water. Therefore, it is recommended that you have a stash of water and portable edibles in your house or car in case of emergencies. Portable edibles should include food that doesn't melt easily in the heat and will resist spoilage. These foods could include:

+ Granola bars

+ Trail mix

+ Nuts

+ Hard, dry cheeses (cheddar, Swiss, or Pecorino Romano)

+ Hard breads (bagels)

+ Vacuum-sealed meat (chicken, tuna, jerky)

+ Canned beans

+ Hard candies

+ Drink mixes

TRAINING AND CERTIFICATION CLASSES

It's also a good idea to have some formal first aid training. Formalized classes offer hands-on experience when it comes to identifying and treating medical emergencies. The good news is, most are offered at low cost or free and are held by organizations all over your city. Seek out your local fire department, police department, and hospital. Inquire about classes through the Red Cross, Salvation Army, local church groups, social groups, civic groups, community-based organizations, parks and recreation departments, and so on.

The following recommended training and or certification classes will make you better prepared to aid in an emergency. Not all are required, and some may be just interesting rather than practical, but you can never learn too much.

+ Cardiopulmonary resuscitation (CPR)

+ Automated external defibrillator (AED)

+ First aid

+ Emergency medical technician (EMT)

+ Blood-borne pathogen awareness

+ Wilderness first aid

+ Specific medical emergency treatment (diabetes, seizure disorder, etc.)

+ Herbal medicine

+ Outdoor survival

+ Stress management

+ PTSD awareness and treatment

+ Physical fitness training

SMARTPHONE APPS

With advances in technology, we're never too far removed from anyone or anything. Seemingly limitless information is at our fingertips or only as far away as our pocket or purse. And while a reliance on technology can be dangerous—such as in the event of a natural disaster, when we may not have cellular access—it can also be a useful tool. Apps and books can be downloaded onto a smartphone or tablet and be accessed at any time, even without a cell signal. Then, you're only limited by the life of the battery and the ability or inability to recharge it. The following list contains recommended apps that you should consider downloading to your device for quick access at times when you need it most.

Recommended apps:

+ **Flashlight**: uses your camera flash to cast light

+ **Compass**: can be used to determine direction and coordinates

+ **Dropbox**: a file-hosting service that can store copies of many important personal documents, as well as maps, checklists, and even books

+ **Pocket first aid**: a compact but thorough first aid guide

+ **Pocket first aid and CPR**: a first aid guide inclusive of CPR procedures

+ **Pet first aid**: a first aid guide for household pets

+ **SAS Survival Guide**: a popular and all-inclusive survival guide that can be downloaded onto your device

+ **iMap Weather Radio**: a handy, easy-to-operate weather radio

+ **Google Maps**: a useful mapping tool to use if you have a cellular signal

+ **Google Earth**: similar to Google Maps, and also requires a cellular signal

+ **Skype**: free Web-based video calling service

+ **The Weather Channel**: allows you to stay in tune with the latest weather forecast

+ **Red Panic Button**: allows you to send prewritten or custom messages to predetermined people via text or email

+ **FEMA**: offers weather alerts, safety tips, maps, and additional assistance

+ **Life 360**: location sharing among family and friends

+ **Backcountry Navigator**: outdoor navigation app featuring topographic maps and GPS

CHAPTER 2

CONTROLLING BLOOD LOSS

Whether it's in the moments following a disaster or somewhere out in the wild, the most common injury that will require treatment is bleeding. Controlling blood loss can be as simple as applying an adhesive bandage to cover a scrape, or as critical as administering a tourniquet in order to save a life. The one thing you can be sure of is that in most emergency situations there will be a large number of injuries that are going to require some type of bleeding control.

There are some things that you should know about blood loss and the human body. First of all, blood loss can be deceiving. Blood has a tendency to spread itself very thin, creating massive pools that give the appearance of major loss when in reality it could be a small amount. People have an urgent reaction to blood and feel the need to "fix" it immediately, but because people come in such a wide variety of sizes and shapes, there is no set amount of blood that a person can lose before it becomes dangerous. The U.S. Air Force's *Self Aid and Buddy Care Instructor Handbook* states that a person has an average of 5 to 6 liters of blood in their body, although that number will vary slightly depending on the person. As a general rule, you can assume that at 40 percent blood loss, bad things can begin to happen to a patient. But the reality is, how are you to know? You have no realistic way of determining whether a person has lost 30 percent of their blood or 50 percent.

The body has built-in defense mechanisms that will help stop bleeding once it has begun. Hemostasis is the process that causes bleeding to stop.

The blood vessels restrict, platelets stick together to cover the break in the vessel wall, and the blood begins to clot. When the wound is too great for hemostasis to stop the bleeding, other measures must be taken.

TYPES OF BLEEDING

There are three types of external bleeding, each with a different degree of seriousness.

Capillary: Capillaries are the smallest blood vessels in your body. When they're cut open, it usually leads to slow-oozing blood that is easily controllable. Hemostasis is able to stop this bleeding in most cases.

Venous: Venous blood is blood that is returning to the heart by way of the veins. Deeper, more invasive cuts have the potential to cut veins that will typically lead to more significant bleeding than capillary bleeding. The blood will be a dark red or maroon color, and the bleeding is often controlled by applying direct pressure.

Arterial: Arterial bleeding is the most serious, yet fortunately the least common. Arteries are vessels that are carrying oxygenated blood away from the heart. A cut artery is characterized by bright red blood that often spurts in time with the beat of the heart. A large amount of blood loss is common with a cut artery because blood in arteries is under pressure. Quick action must be taken in the case of arterial bleeding. If not, it can quickly become fatal.

TYPES OF TREATMENT

DIRECT PRESSURE AND ELEVATION

The most common and simplest way to control blood loss is to apply direct pressure. In fact, most people never have to be taught this. Instinctively, when faced with a break in the skin, people will cover it. What many don't realize is what happens in the body while they're just trying to "plug the hole": They're assisting the hemostasis process. Holding direct pressure stops or slows the bleeding, allowing the platelets to stick together and blood to clot.

Remove or cut any clothing so you have a full view of the wound. Modesty should be considered and protected when possible. There's no need to expose more of the patient than necessary, but it is also important to see what you are working with and to have access to the source of the bleeding. Also, swelling is often an issue, so jewelry in close proximity to the wound should be removed and kept with the patient.

With a gloved hand (a bare hand should only be used as a last resort), hold sterile gauze against the wound. While sterile gauze is obviously preferred, in many situations you'll have to make do with what you have available— often a tattered shirt or other cloth. The cleanest fabric you can find will give you the best chance to stop the bleeding while trying to prevent infection.

Hold direct pressure over the entire wound for a minimum of 15 minutes. Avoid the urge to remove the bandage to check to see if bleeding has stopped. By doing that, you interrupt the clotting process. Fifteen minutes will seem like a long time, but it should allow enough time for the body's internal process to stop or at least slow the bleeding. If blood soaks through the bandage during that time, do not replace it; instead, place more bandages over the existing bandage. Occasionally, there may be an object in the wound. If that is the case, apply pressure around the wound without pressing directly on the object.

Gravity can be a useful tool when you're attempting to stop any kind of bleeding. Think back to when you were in school and raised your hand to ask a question. If the teacher didn't call on you right away, your arm began to tire and your fingers would start to tingle. You would switch arms and begin the process over. The tingling was caused by poor circulation. Your heart was struggling to pump blood against gravity. If it is possible and doesn't cause further pain for the patient, hold pressure on the wound and elevate it above the heart. Gravity will help reduce blood loss.

In the case of a mass-casualty incident when you have limited resources to aid a large number of patients, those requiring direct-pressure wound care can help treat themselves and each other. Unless there are other, more severe medical issues, a patient requiring direct pressure to a wound can often apply the pressure to themselves and/or others, freeing you up to treat additional victims.

The *US Army Survival Manual* dictates:

> *If bleeding continues after having applied direct pressure for 30 minutes, apply a pressure dressing. This dressing consists of a thick dressing of gauze or other suitable material applied directly over the wound and held in place with a tightly wrapped bandage. It should be tighter than an ordinary compression bandage but not so tight that it impairs circulation to the rest of the limb. Once you apply the dressing, do not remove it, even when the dressing becomes blood soaked.*

PRESSURE POINTS

The vast majority of the time, direct pressure and elevation will control bleeding. The next step is to apply force to a pressure point, which will reduce circulation to an area of the body. By reducing the blood flow to a specific area, you effectively diminish the amount of blood that *can* be lost. Pressure points are found in all parts of the body, but are most commonly used in treating the extremities.

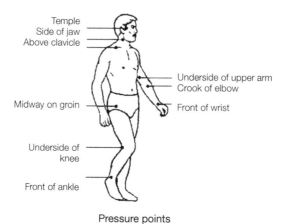

Pressure points

Pressure points are actually arteries where, by applying pressure, you can greatly reduce the amount of blood being circulated to the injury. (An artery pumps oxygenated blood from the heart throughout the body.) Pressing the artery against a bone is like putting a kink in a garden hose. You should note, however, that there are inherent risks to restricting blood flow. If you inadvertently stop the blood flow altogether, you run the risk of necrosis in the area beyond the restriction. Necrosis is the death of cells due to the lack of oxygenated blood. As a general rule, you should not restrict blood flow for more than 10 minutes. If a patient has suffered an injury significant enough to require the use of pressure points, they should receive advanced care as soon as possible.

Although pressure points are located throughout the body, some are more dangerous than others to utilize, such as the carotid artery, located in the neck. The arteries most commonly used to restrict blood flow are the brachial, radial, femoral, and popliteal. These are most easily located on the underside of the upper arm, the front of the wrist, midway on the groin, and the underside of the knee, respectively.

TOURNIQUET

A tourniquet is the third and last resort to stop severe bleeding. Using the same principle as pressure points, a tourniquet utilizes a band or strip of cloth to even further restrict blood flow. Tourniquets are commonly used to bring veins to the surface when you are giving blood or receiving an IV. The health-care provider wraps an elastic band around your biceps and then locates a vein for cannulation ("cannulation" roughly means a tube being inserted into the body, such as an IV needle).

Some first aid kits may provide a tourniquet, but for the most part, they are primarily used by hospital staff, paramedics, and military personnel, rather than the general public. It has long been believed that applying a tourniquet is a risky maneuver that can lead to further injury to the victim, and for decades the practice had fallen out of favor in first aid. Recently, however, studies are showing that even tourniquets that are not applied exactly correctly can still make a positive difference when utilized in the field. A 2009 study conducted by the U.S. Army Institute of Surgical Research set out to determine if emergency tourniquet use saved lives, and the answer was an overwhelming yes.

To apply a tourniquet, you must first select the right material. Tactical tourniquets are issued to military medical personnel to keep in their medical supply kits. There are many military-grade tourniquets on the market available to the general public, and they are relatively inexpensive and come with complete instructions. In a disaster situation, however, you may not have access to a premade tourniquet kit and will be forced to improvise. Use the following steps to administer a tourniquet:

1. Use a piece of cloth or elastic band, preferably 1 to 2 inches wide.

2. Place it 2 to 4 inches away from the wound toward the core of the body.

3. Use padding underneath the tourniquet to avoid cutting into the skin.

4. Tie a half-knot (the same knot used as the first part of tying your shoe).

5. Place a stick (or similar rigid object) on top of the half-knot.

6. Tie a full-knot over the stick.

7. Twist the stick until the tourniquet is tight around the limb and the bleeding has stopped. Blood may ooze for a short time, and this is to be expected.

8. Fasten the tourniquet to the injured limb in a way that prevents it from loosening by 1) applying the tie two inches above the wound, 2) inserting the stick, 3), turning the stick until the bleeding is controlled, and 4) securing the stick.

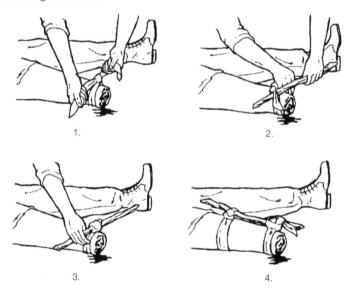

Warning: Applying direct pressure and locating pressure points are the best options to help prevent blood loss. They are the easiest to perform and offer the least chance for complications. Only in the direst of circumstances should a tourniquet to be considered.

CLOTTING AGENTS

Clotting agents have been successfully used in the military for years and have found their way into common use in emergency medicine. A clotting agent is a medical treatment used to control severe bleeding that can come as a gel, powder, or pretreated gauze dressing. The dressing is impregnated with kaolin (or something similar), a mineral that accelerates the body's natural clotting process. The most commonly used clotting agents, such as QuikClot, Celox, and HemCon, all work on a three-minute "hold in place" model, so despite a common misconception, clotting doesn't occur instantly.

A clotting agent is most often used when the number of patients or conditions doesn't allow for slow, methodical treatment. The powder version is becoming less commonly used in favor of the treated dressing, which can be packed into a wound and dissolves over time as the body heals itself. Be it on the battlefield or following a disastrous event that has resulted in many casualties, a clotting agent can be a big asset. It has the ability to rapidly control bleeding, which alone can be the difference between the victim becoming a survivor or a casualty, and it quickly frees you up to treat other patients.

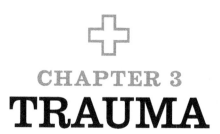

CHAPTER 3
TRAUMA

Physical trauma comes in many forms. It is defined as "an injury (as a wound) to living tissue caused by an extrinsic agent." Basically, it is an outside force acting upon the body that causes an injury. Examples are all around us: car wrecks, falls, explosions, gunshots, and blunt and penetrating injuries. According to the National Trauma Institute, trauma accounts for 47 percent of deaths from ages 1 to 46, which makes it the number one cause of death in that age group and the number three cause of death across all age groups.

A traumatic injury can be fatal even under the best of circumstances. I once responded to an injury accident that was literally in front of one of our local hospitals that happened to be one of two trauma centers in the area. A man swerved his motorcycle to avoid a car, ended up hitting the curb, and was thrown to the ground. We quickly loaded him into the ambulance and rushed him to the emergency room, which was about a stone's throw from the accident, where unfortunately he succumbed to his injuries. Short of crashing a motorcycle *into* an ER, you can't get much closer than that man was, and the trauma he sustained still proved to be fatal.

Without exception, the best treatment you can offer someone who has experienced physical trauma of any kind is getting them to a hospital as soon as possible. There is very little field treatment you can offer someone who has internal injuries. But when you're in the wilderness or any other kind of survival situation where advanced care is not an immediate option, you need to know what your treatment options are for various traumatic injuries.

TYPES OF TRAUMA AND INITIAL TREATMENT OBJECTIVES

There are four main types of trauma: blunt force trauma, falling, gunshot, and stabbing/impalement. Your trauma treatment objectives are:

1. **Recognition**: Identify, as best you can, the extent of injuries, especially those that may be life-threatening.

2. **Treatment**: Initiate supportive therapy. Do the best you can for the patient with what you have available.

3. **Transport**: Transfer the injured person to a location (typically a hospital) that can provide definitive treatment.

BLUNT FORCE TRAUMA

Severe trauma to the body or head with the sudden introduction of a blunt instrument used with great force is blunt force trauma. Put another way, it's when you're hit with something or by someone. It can be as benign as the bruise left when one brother punches another in the arm, or as dangerous as crossing the street and getting hit by a bus. It can come from a fist, a baseball bat, a vehicle, or anything that can cause injury when it quickly impacts the body.

Often the effects of blunt force trauma aren't immediately visible. If a laceration cuts or tears the skin, there can be varying degrees of bleeding, but often the danger with blunt force trauma occurs inside the body. As taught in the U.S. Air Force's *Self Aid and Buddy Care Instructor Handbook*, there are signs and symptoms you can identify both internally and externally.

Signs and Symptoms

Bruising: Broken blood vessels below the surface of the skin are what we see as a bruise. Bruising should not be taken as an indicator of the severity of the injury. There can also be significant bruising deeper inside the body that isn't visible, sometimes to vital organs. Bruising should be used to identify a specific location where trauma occurred, but not as a gauge of how bad an injury is.

Abrasions: Harsh grazing of the skin can cause abrasions. An abrasion is a superficial injury to the outer layer of skin (epidermis) and, like bruising, is a mark of where trauma occurred, but not a gauge of its severity. Often abrasions occur when someone is dragged or during a fall.

Lacerations: A laceration is a deep cut or tearing of the skin. Lacerations can be deadly depending on their depth and location. External lacerations are obvious due to the telltale bleeding, but a more common result of blunt force trauma is an internal laceration. Like external lacerations, an internal laceration can lead to death, depending on which organ was impacted and how severely.

Treatment

Any or all of the above could be indicators of blunt force trauma, but none has to be present to show that it occurred. The biggest concern is internal injuries, and because the injuries are often internal, there isn't much treatment that can be done other than bleeding control (see Chapter 2) and fracture management (see Chapter 5). Again, it's worth repeating that anytime you suspect blunt force trauma, you should transport the victim to a hospital as soon as possible. In a disaster situation, when taking the victim to a hospital is not an option, your goal in treating the patient is to make them comfortable and ensure they maintain their ABCs (see page 20). There is little that can be done in the field for what are likely internal injuries.

FALLING

Falling is dangerous at any age and from any height. At my fire department, Engine 44 Captain Pat DuPont once told me, "A fall from anything above the third floor is interesting only," meaning it doesn't take a large distance for a fall to be fatal, and beyond a certain height, the outcome is almost always the same. But the other end of the spectrum can also be true. As we age, our bones become more brittle, and even falling from a standing position can be extremely dangerous. Many medical protocols consider any fall from greater than 10 feet to be a "long fall," which moves the patient into another level of trauma classification.

Regardless of the height, there are specific injuries that are inherent to falls: head injuries, spinal injuries, broken bones, and torn tendons and ligaments.

Signs and Symptoms

The signs and symptoms of a fall are often evident. If the person is conscious, they can tell you what hurts, where, and how badly. Sometimes you can see an obvious fracture and treat the injury. However, there is also the chance of internal injuries, which can be the bigger concern. When someone has suffered a fall, they should be checked head to toe for fractures, a head injury, or any other associated issues in the following signs and symptoms:

+ Obvious fractures

+ Localized pain

+ Bleeding

+ Nausea/vomiting

+ Weakness

+ Headache

+ Slurred speech

+ Loss of motor function

+ Numbness/tingling

+ Unequal pupils

+ Loss of consciousness

Treatment

1. Stabilize the spine. If you have another person to assist you, have them perform spinal stabilization while you continue with your assessment.

To stabilize a spine, you hold the patient's head in the same position in which you found it, as long as the patient is able to breathe in this position. Keep any movement of the patient to a minimum. If the patient is conscious, you may need to reassure them and explain that they should keep still and do their best to remain calm and relaxed.

2. Ensure the patient has their ABCs.

3. Perform a head-to-toe assessment, identifying and prioritizing injuries.

4. Stop significant bleeding.

5. Immobilize fractures.

6. Monitor the status of the patient and injuries.

GUNSHOT

A sad fact is that there has been as sharp rise in civil disturbances and public active shooter incidents in the United States over the last decade. Battlefields, which were once in news stories about faraway places, are now in our schools and shopping malls. The purpose of this section is not to take a stance for or against guns, it is to address the problems that occur as a result of a gunshot wound. When faced with a patient who has experienced a gunshot wound, it is particularly important to assess scene safety before rendering aid.

Signs and Symptoms

+ Open wound at the entrance site

+ Open wound if there is an exit site (there isn't always an exit wound)

+ Bleeding

+ Pain

+ Possible loss of consciousness

Treatment

General treatment for a gunshot wound rearranges the ABC acronym to CAB, placing "circulation" first. Often when dealing with a gunshot wound, the primary issue is circulation and, regardless of the airway, the wound must be addressed first. *The Special Operation Forces Medical Handbook* details what to do in the event of a gunshot wound. The following are steps that are appropriate for non-surgically trained responders to perform.

1. **Expose the wound**: Typically with gunshots, there are two wounds for every projectile: an entrance wound and an exit wound. While protecting the patient's modesty as best you can, you should expose as much of the body as possible. Bullets can enter the body and ricochet, so an exit wound can be far away from the entrance wound. It is best to be able to examine the entire body and then cover any area where you don't need to administer aid.

2. Control bleeding: Use direct pressure and elevation first. For more serious bleeding consider using pressure points, a tourniquet, or a clotting agent.

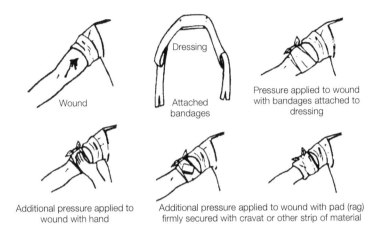

How to apply field dressings to wounds

3. Treat for shock: Although there has been some debate recently over the effectiveness of patient positioning, you should still place the person in the Trendelenburg position. (The Trendelenburg position is placing the victim on their back at an angle by elevating their pelvis and legs above the heart.) Cover the patient for warmth and administer oxygen if you have it available.

Do not attempt to locate the bullet and remove it. It is often fragmented or buried so deep within the body that you'll do more harm than good trying to locate it. There are thousands of military veterans who live with bullets or shrapnel in their bodies. The body can sometimes adapt with very few complications.

Considerations for Specific Gunshot Injuries

Extremities: bleeding control, swelling (which could be a sign of internal bleeding), and broken bones

As you control bleeding, watch for swelling, and if you suspect a bone fracture, splint appropriately.

Chest: bleeding control, treat open or "sucking" chest wound (so named because it can allow air into the lungs leading to lung collapse), take spinal precautions, and be aware that vital organ damage is likely.

Control bleeding and cover any sucking chest wound with an occlusive dressing. Hold the patient's head to prevent neck and spinal movement, and seek advanced care as soon as possible.

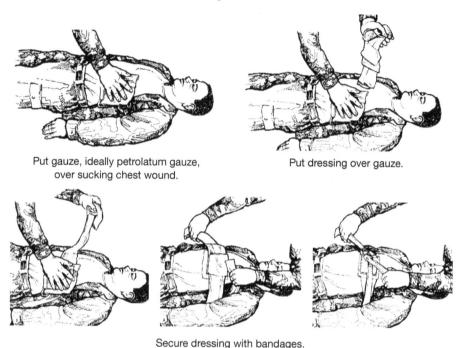

Put gauze, ideally petrolatum gauze, over sucking chest wound.

Put dressing over gauze.

Secure dressing with bandages.

Head: bleeding control, protect the airway, seek advanced care

Direct pressure and elevation are really the only practical methods to control bleeding from a gunshot wound to the head in the field. If the victim is conscious, you can have them sit up and lean forward. If the person is unconscious, the best way to protect the airway is to turn them on their side and bend their top knee forward to help keep them in that position.

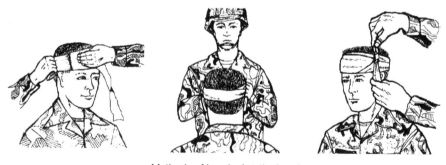

Methods of bandaging the head

STABBING/IMPALEMENT

A stabbing, whether it occurred intentionally or unintentionally, should be treated the same as any impalement injury, just as any impalement should be treated as a stabbing. It could be the result of an assault, a fall, an explosion, or any other type of violent scenario. To avoid becoming a victim as well, only approach the patient once you have determined it is safe to do so.

Impalement injuries can be complicated because not only can they cause significant blood loss, but there is almost always internal trauma that cannot be treated in the field. There is also a high chance for infection. Whether it is stitches or surgery, there is nearly always the need for advanced care, so transport the patient to a hospital or trauma center as soon as possible.

Treatment

Superficial and minor stab wounds can be treated with general first aid, but anything more invasive is beyond the scope of the layperson performing field medicine. If a more significant stabbing or impalement occurs, perform the following steps:

1. **Determine scene safety and put on your PPE (minimum of gloves and eye protection).**

    + Inspect the patient to determine the extent of their injuries. It is possible, particularly after an explosion or an assault, that the patient will have multiple wounds that will require treatment. Locate all the wounds, determine if any are potentially life-threatening, and prioritize which are treated first.

    + Talk with the victim (if they are conscious) and reassure them. You can try to take their mind off the injury with conversation. If the knife or other foreign object is still in the body, you should cover it, or keep the person from being able to see it.

    + DO NOT remove any objects that are impaled in the body. Once an object has been forced into the body, the trauma has occurred, and removing it could create even more trauma. Sometimes the impaled object is actually helping to stem the blood flow, reducing the amount of blood lost. It is best to somehow support the object so that it doesn't wiggle around or get bumped, causing more damage. If an eye is impaled, before stabilizing the impaled object, you should cover the unaffected eye. Eyes tend to move together and by covering the unaffected eye, you're better able to keep the impaled eye still and stable.

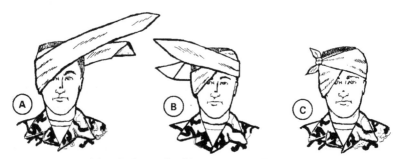

A bandaging method to cover an unaffected eye
while leaving the impaled eye free to stabilize

+ Treat the most significant bleeding first. ABCs are always the medical priorities, but with impalement, blood loss poses the greatest threat that can be treated in the field. Locate all wounds and identify which will require the most immediate treatment. Utilize direct pressure and elevation when possible, followed by pressure points, and then a tourniquet.

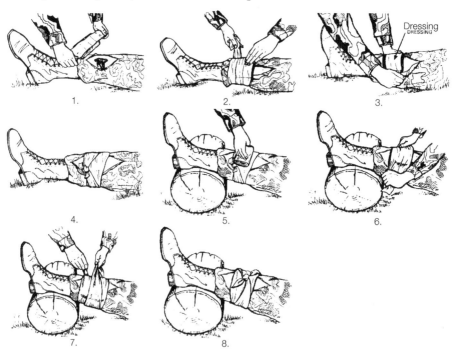

Example of a leg wound bandaged and elevated

+ Once bleeding is managed, clean the wounds. Even if wounds don't appear to have debris, they should be cleaned, because whatever created them was likely not sterile. There are very effective over-the-counter products that are used for cleaning wounds, but clean water can be used to irrigate a wound. Be sure to warn the patient before you do, though, because irrigating a wound can be surprising and painful.

2. **Close wounds that you are able to**. Adhesive bandages can be used for superficial wounds. For larger wounds use butterfly bandages; it's also possible to use superglue or duct tape if needed. If you have antibiotic ointment available, apply it once the wound is cleaned and closed.

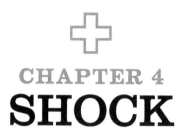

CHAPTER 4
SHOCK

The term "shock" is thrown around rather recklessly in the area of medical aid. There's a difference between psychological shock and medical shock, but "shock" is often used as a generic catch-all for someone who has been adversely affected by an event when a specific medical diagnosis can't be assigned. Psychological shock will be discussed in Chapter 15.

Medical shock (also known as physiological shock) occurs when tissue and organs don't receive an adequate flow of blood to function normally. When there's a lack of oxygenated blood, a buildup of waste occurs and creates a condition known as shock, which can be caused by many different things such as an allergic reaction, blood loss, or severe infection. Basically, shock is when, for whatever reason, blood flow or blood volume is not sufficient to meet the body's needs. Shock can be a dangerous, even life-threatening, condition and can lead to hypoxia (a lack of oxygen in the body's tissue), organ damage, and cardiac arrest.

One important thing to keep in mind is that "shock" is not an actual diagnosis. It's a symptom of a bigger problem that requires medical attention as soon as possible. The patient's condition can rapidly worsen, so immediate treatment is necessary. The U.S. Air Force's *Self Aid and Buddy Care Instructor Handbook* explains, "Shock stuns and weakens the body. When the normal blood flow in the body is upset, death can result. Early identification and proper treatment may save the casualty's life."

FOUR STAGES OF SHOCK

1. **Initial stage**: Typically, there are no signs and symptoms at this stage. The body is just beginning to feel that something is wrong. Cells are beginning to change due to complications with perfusion (the delivery of oxygenated blood to the organs, muscle, and tissue). This stage is reversible, but difficult to identify because most changes occur internally.

2. **Compensatory stage**: At this point, the body has identified that something is wrong and it begins to take action to compensate. Hyperventilation is an example of what may occur. The body recognizes that it isn't receiving adequate oxygen, so it will automatically increase respiration, attempting to compensate for the deficit. When blood pressure begins to drop, the adrenal glands secrete a hormone that will increase the heart rate in an attempt to compensate for low blood pressure. Something is wrong, and the body is doing what it can to fix it.

3. **Progressive stage**: At this stage, cellular function deteriorates and organ damage may begin. The damage at this point may be irreversible.

4. **Refractory stage**: If the cause of shock cannot be fixed, the body will enter the final stage of shock: organ failure and death. The goal of treating shock is to prevent the patient from reaching these dire outcomes.

SIGNS AND SYMPTOMS OF GENERAL SHOCK

In situations where we may not know the specific cause of shock, there are general symptoms the patient may be feeling that will help us identify that shock may be occurring so we can begin treatment.

Early Symptoms:

+ Cool/sweaty skin

+ Rapid pulse

+ Anxiety

Late Symptoms:

+ Weakness/dizziness

+ Nausea/vomiting

+ Rapid/shallow breathing

+ Confusion

+ Thirst

+ Weakening pulse

+ Blue lips and fingernails (cyanosis)

+ Loss of consciousness

The following sections discuss specific types of shock, along with their associated signs and symptoms. Remember that not *all* signs and symptoms need to be present. Listed are things you may expect to see.

ANAPHYLACTIC SHOCK

Anaphylaxis, or anaphylactic shock, is a severe allergic reaction that can be caused by something the patient has ingested such as food or drink, medical tools such as latex or penicillin, or other allergens like bee or wasp stings. See page 85 for more information on anaphylaxis.

Signs and Symptoms

+ Dizziness

+ Loss of consciousness

+ Labored breathing

+ Swelling of the tongue

+ Blue lips and fingernails (cyanosis)

+ Low blood pressure (hypotension)

+ Heart failure

CARDIOGENIC SHOCK

Cardiogenic shock occurs when the heart has been severely damaged, often by a heart attack.

Signs and Symptoms

+ Rapid breathing

+ Severe shortness of breath

+ Sudden, rapid heartbeat (tachycardia)

+ Loss of consciousness

+ Weak pulse

+ Sweating

+ Pale skin

+ Cold hands or feet

+ Urinating less than normal or not at all

HYPOVOLEMIC SHOCK

Hypovolemic shock (or hemorrhagic shock) occurs when the body's total blood volume drops to a dangerous level that can be caused by internal or external bleeding, dehydration, or disease, among other things. Blood loss leading to hypovolemic shock is a major concern in military operations. The *US Army Survival Manual* tells us to anticipate shock in all battlefield injuries.

Signs and Symptoms

+ External bleeding

+ Anxiety

+ Blue lips and fingernails (cyanosis)

+ Low or no urine output

+ Profuse sweating

+ Shallow breathing

+ Dizziness

+ Light-headedness

+ Confusion

+ Chest pain

+ Loss of consciousness

+ Low blood pressure (hypotension)

+ Rapid heart rate (tachycardia)

+ Weak pulse

It is more difficult to recognize hypovolemic shock if the patient's bleeding is all internal. However, there are still signs and symptoms to indicate what is wrong.

Signs and Symptoms

+ Abdominal pain

+ Blood in the stool

+ Black, tarry stool (melena)

+ Blood in the urine

+ Vaginal bleeding (heavy and outside of normal menstruation)

+ Vomiting blood

+ Chest pain

+ Abdominal swelling

NEUROGENIC SHOCK

Neurogenic shock is when there is a disruption of the automatic pathways within the spinal cord. It often follows an injury to the central nervous system, such as a spinal injury.

Signs and Symptoms

+ Low blood pressure (hypotension)

+ Low heart rate (bradycardia)

SEPTIC SHOCK

Septic shock is a widespread inflammatory response to infection. It occurs when blood becomes toxic due to a bacterial infection.

Signs and Symptoms

+ Significantly decreased urine output

+ Abrupt change in mental status

+ Decrease in platelet count

+ Difficulty breathing

+ Abnormal heart pumping function

+ Abdominal pain

GENERAL SHOCK TREATMENT

The key to treating shock is early recognition. Once you recognize the signs and symptoms and understand that there is a bigger issue at hand, you can begin to treat the victim. The *US Army Survival Manual* outlines the steps for treating shock:

+ Lie the victim on their back.

+ Ensure their ABCs.

+ Control bleeding if necessary.

+ Elevate the feet 6 to 12 inches.

+ Loosen clothing.

+ Provide cooling or warmth to make the victim comfortable.

Conscious victim

+ Place on a level surface

+ Remove all wet clothing

+ Give warm fluids

+ Insulate from the ground

+ Shelter from weather

+ Maintain body heat

+ Elevate lower extremities 15 to 20 cm (6 to 8 in)

+ Allow at least 24 hours rest

Unconscious victim

Same as for conscious victim except:

+ Place victim on side and turn head to one side to prevent choking on vomit, blood, or other fluids

+ Do not elevate extremities

+ Do not administer fluids

✚

CHAPTER 5

FRACTURES

After bleeding, bone fractures are the second most frequent type of injury that you may have to treat when you are beyond the reach of immediate emergency help. Fractures are extremely common, and although they can be life-threatening, in many cases they are very manageable. One common issue that responders encounter both on the battlefield and at emergency scenes are fractures that become a *distracting injury*, or an injury that draws attention away from less obvious, more life-threatening issues. For example, someone may have a disfigured, broken arm and be screaming in pain, bringing attention to the visually disturbing injury, while they are quietly succumbing to an unnoticed head wound. So while fractures must be addressed, don't allow them to distract from other injuries.

As with bleeding, a fracture's visual appearance may not reflect actual severity. The injury may not be as severe as it looks; likewise, it can be worse. Once treated, the injury should be out of the patient's sight if possible. Once, I was off-duty and attending my son's football game when players began to yell and scatter at the end of a play. Members of the crowd began to gasp. I finally noticed what the commotion was about. One of the players was on his back, knees up, and his right leg at the shin was twisted and flopped to the side with his foot facing backward. Even from the stands it was an obvious tibia/fibula compound fracture. The trainers ran to the field. Typically, I leave treatment to the capable men and women who are trained to be there, but because of the severity of the injury and my knowledge that the responding ambulance was still far away, I went down to the field to offer assistance.

The trainers had the ice and splints that would be needed to help him. My only contribution was advising them to splint it in place while moving it as little as possible and applying ice. I then asked them to cover the injury up so the player wouldn't be able to see it. I held his hand, letting him squeeze mine, assured him that he was OK, and distracted him with conversation. Soon his screaming stopped and, while he was still in pain, he was answering my questions about how their season was going and who his favorite football player was. By splinting, removing the visual, and talking to him in a calming manner, we were able to make the best of a bad situation until help arrived.

The overall objective of fracture management is bleeding control, pain relief, prevention of an ischemia-perfusion injury (when blood supply to an area of tissue is cut off), and removal of potential sources of contamination.

SIGNS AND SYMPTOMS

The signs and symptoms of a fracture are:

+ Pain

+ Tenderness

+ Discoloration

+ Swelling

+ Deformity

+ Loss of function

+ Grating (a sound or feeling that occurs when broken bone ends rub together)

TYPES OF FRACTURES

The *US Army Survival Manual* states that there are two types of fractures: open and closed.

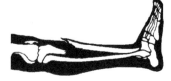

Open: With an open (or compound) fracture, the bone protrudes through the skin and complicates the actual fracture with an open wound. In a survival situation, someone who has been trained to do so may consider setting the fracture. However, unless you are trained in this practice, you should avoid it. Significant complications can arise if it is done incorrectly. You should splint the fracture and treat the wound as any other open wound.

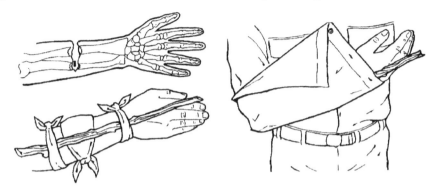

Dressing and improvised splint on open fracture (more rigid material and more ties if available)

Jacket used as improvised sling

Closed: The closed fracture has no open wounds. Follow the guidelines for immobilization (see page 59), and set (if trained to do so) and splint the fracture.

The dangers with any fracture are the severing or the compression of a nerve or blood vessel at the site of the fracture. For this reason, there should be minimum manipulation of the fracture site, and any manipulation should 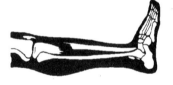 be done very cautiously. If you notice the area below the break becoming numb, swollen, cool to the touch, or turning pale, and the victim shows signs of shock, there is likely a problem with circulation, or a major vessel may have been severed.

TREATMENT

EXTREMITY FRACTURES

For treating an extremity fracture, perform the following procedures:

1. Evaluate the patient: Be prepared to perform any necessary lifesaving measures. Monitor the patient for development of conditions that may require you to perform such measures.

2. **Locate the site of the suspected fracture**: Ask the patient for the location of the injury.

+ Does the patient have any pain?
  * Where is it tender?
  * Can they move the extremity?

With the presence of an obvious deformity, do not make the patient move the extremity. Movement will be extremely painful and could further the injury. Observe the extremity's fracture for an unnatural position. Look for a bone sticking out (protruding).

3. **Prepare the patient for splinting the fracture**:

+ Reassure the patient. Tell them that you will be providing first aid and that you will get them medical help as soon as possible. Loosen any tight or binding clothing.

+ Remove all jewelry from the injured area and place it in the patient's pocket. It's always a good idea to tell the patient why you are removing jewelry and assure them that you will put it in their pocket or purse, or give it to a trusted acquaintance of the patient.

+ Gather splinting materials. If standard splinting materials (splints, padding, and ties) are not available, gather improvised materials.

+ Pad the splints where they touch any bony part of the body, such as the elbow, wrist, knee, ankle, crotch, or armpit. Padding prevents excessive pressure on the area, which could lead to circulation problems.

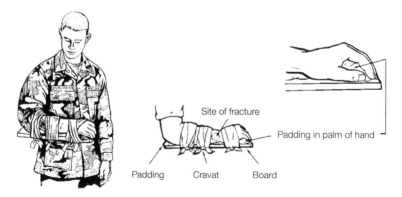

Cravats placed above and below fracture with knots tied against board

Cravat cradles knee: Cravat is placed around the splint, between the boards under the knee, thus cradling the knee (the knee protrudes above the splints)

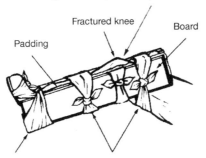

Fractured knee

Board

Padding

Cravat to secure ankle (cupped under heel, crossed on top of boot, crossed on sole of boot, tied on top of boot)

Cravats placed above and below fracture, knots tied against board

+ Check circulation below the site of the injury. Note any pale, white, or bluish-gray color of the skin, which may indicate impaired circulation. Circulation can also be checked by performing a blanch test—depressing the toenail or fingernail beds and observing how quickly the color returns. A slower return of color to the injured side when compared with the uninjured side indicates a problem with circulation. The fingernail bed is the method to use to check the circulation in a dark-skinned patient.

+ Check the temperature of the injured extremity. Use your hand to compare the temperature of the injured side with the uninjured side. The body area below the injury may be colder to the touch, indicating poor circulation.

+ Question the patient about the presence of numbness, tightness, cold, or tingling sensations.

4. **Immobilize the injury**:

+ Apply the splint in place. Splint the fracture in the position found. DO NOT attempt to reposition or straighten the injury.

+ If it is an open fracture, stop the bleeding and protect the wound. Cover all wounds with field dressings before applying a splint. Place one splint on each side of the fracture. Make sure that the splints reach, if possible, beyond the joints above and below the fracture.

+ Tie the splints. Secure each splint in place above and below the fracture site with fabric that can be used to tie. Improvised ties such as strips of cloth, belts, or whatever else you have may be used. With minimal motion to the injured areas, place and tie the splints with the bandages. Push ties through and under the natural body curvatures, and then gently position the fabric and tie in place. Use square knots. DO NOT tie directly over the suspected fracture site. Check for tightness. Be sure that bandages are tight enough to securely hold the splinting materials in place, but not so tight that circulation is impaired.

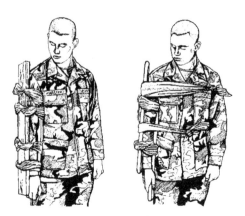

5. Recheck the circulation after application of the splint:

Check the skin color and temperature. This is to ensure that the bandages holding the splint in place have not been tied too tightly. A fingertip check can be made by inserting the tip of a finger between the bandaged knot and the skin.

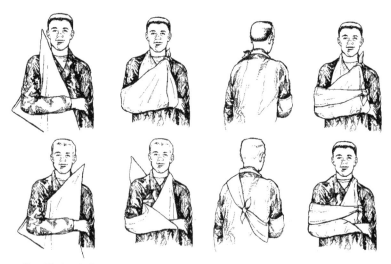

Two kinds of slings that can be used to secure sprains or splinted fractures

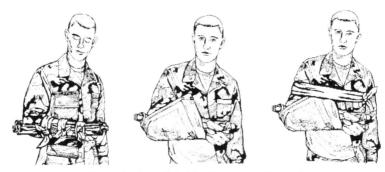

Example of a splinted fracture secured by a sling

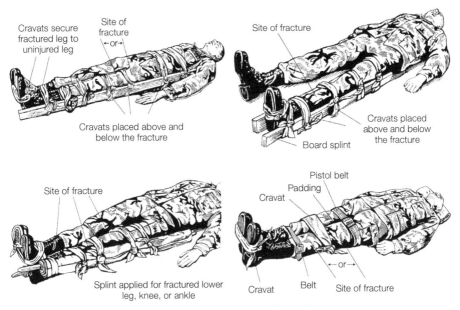

Cravats secure fractured leg to uninjured leg

Site of fracture ←or→

Cravats placed above and below the fracture

Site of fracture

Cravats placed above and below the fracture

Board splint

Site of fracture

Splint applied for fractured lower leg, knee, or ankle

Pistol belt

Padding

Cravat

Cravat

Belt

←or→

Site of fracture

Examples of different kinds of leg splints

Casualties with fractures of the extremities may show impaired circulation, such as numbness and/or tingling, cold, or pale-to-bluish skin. These patients should be evacuated by medical personnel and treated as soon as possible. Prompt medical treatment may prevent possible loss of the limb.

If it is an open fracture and the bone is protruding from the skin, do not attempt to push the bone back under the skin. Apply a field dressing over the wound to protect the area.

OTHER FRACTURES

Extremity fractures are the most common and most easily treatable fractures. Other fractures can be a bit more complicated to treat.

Rib fracture: There is not much that can be done in the field for a rib fracture. It will be extremely painful for the victim. The best thing you can do is minimize movement, make them comfortable, and get them to advanced care.

Skull fracture: The same can be said for skull fractures as rib fractures. The best treatment is to minimize movement and monitor their ABCs. A skull fracture is a very serious injury, and the patient should be given transport priority and evacuated to receive advanced care as soon as possible.

Neck/back fracture: A fractured neck is extremely dangerous. Bone fragments may bruise or cut the spinal cord just as they might in a fractured back. Use caution when moving the patient. Moving may cause permanent injury or death.

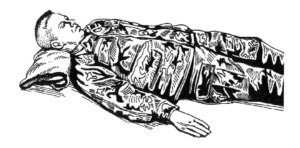

To stabilize a patient with a neck/back fracture, do the following:

1. Leave the patient in the position in which they are found.

2. Keep their head still and in a neutral position, correctly aligned with the neck rather than tilting to one side or the other. If the patient is lying face-up, raise their shoulders slightly, and slip a roll of cloth with the bulk of a bath towel under their neck. If the break is lower, slip the roll of cloth under their lower back.

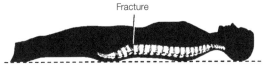

Fracture

In this position, bone fragments may bruise or cut the spinal cord

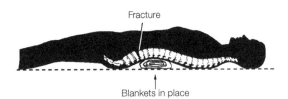

Fracture

Blankets in place

3. If the neck is not in the neutral position, an attempt should be made to achieve alignment. Even if the patient is awake and cooperative, they should allow the rescuer to move their head. If the patient is unconscious or unable to cooperate, simply do it for them. If there is any pain, neurological deterioration, or resistance to movement, the procedure should be abandoned and the neck splinted in the current position.

4. Immobilize the head and neck by gathering heavy objects, such as rocks or the patient's boots filled with dirt, sand, gravel, or rock, and place them on each side of the patient's head. If it is necessary to use boots, tie the tops tightly or stuff with pieces of cloth to secure the contents.

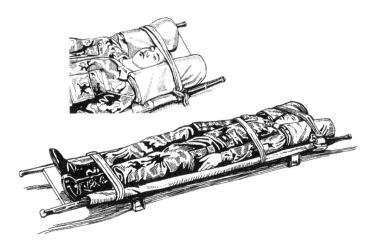

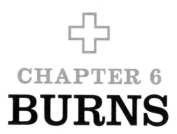

CHAPTER 6
BURNS

Burns are caused by heat, chemicals, electricity, friction, and radiation, and often cause extreme pain, scarring, or even death. In my experience, I've seen all kinds of burns and for all kinds of reasons. Burns are difficult to treat because of the intense pain they cause the patient. For me, the most difficult thing is treating children who have been burned. There is an emotional element when dealing with children, in addition to the physical challenge of trying to get them to follow your instructions and allow you to treat them while they're in great pain. Regardless of the burn victim's age, initial treatment is extremely important to reduce infection and provide pain relief, but the real risk for a burn patient is the infection that follows in the days and weeks after the burn. The *US Army Survival Manual* offers steps to relieve pain, speed healing, and protect against infection, but first you should be able to identify the type of burn.

TYPES OF BURNS

Before administering first aid, you must be able to recognize the type of burn. There are four types of burns:

+ **Electrical burns**: caused by electrical wires, electrical current, or lightning.

+ **Chemical burns**: caused by contact with wet or dry chemicals or white phosphorus (used in illumination and incendiary munitions).

+ **Laser burns**: caused by a device that generates an intense beam of coherent monochromatic light (coherent being that the wavelengths are in phase "waving together").

✛ **Thermal burns**: caused by fire, hot objects, hot liquids, gases, or nuclear blast or fireball

Burn symptoms and treatment are based on the degree of a burn, rather than on its cause. Additional instructions specific to the different types of burns are included below.

Electrical burns: Remove the electrical burn patient from the electrical source by turning off the electrical current. If the shut-off to the source of the electricity is not close by, you may want to quickly consider other options. Speed is critical, so do not waste unnecessary time. If the electricity cannot be turned off, wrap any nonconductive material (dry rope, clothing, wood, and so forth) around the patient's back and shoulders and drag the patient away from the electrical source.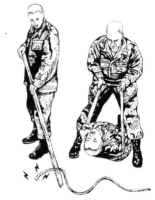
DO NOT make body-to-body contact with the patient or touch any wires, because you too could become an electrical burn casualty.

Chemical burns: Remove the chemical from the burned patient. Remove liquid chemicals by flushing with as much water as possible. Remove dry chemicals by brushing off loose particles (DO NOT use the bare surface of your hand because you too could become a chemical burn casualty) and then flush with large amounts of water, if available. If large amounts of water are not available, then NO water should be applied, because small amounts of water applied to a dry chemical burn may cause a chemical reaction. It should be noted that some chemicals react adversely with water, so it is always best to know what you're dealing with before flushing.

When white phosphorus strikes the skin, smother with a wet cloth or mud. Keep white phosphorus covered with a wet material to keep air out; this should help prevent the particles from burning. Do not lift or cut away clothing from a wound if the patient is still in an environment where the chemical is not contained and is a hazard. Apply the dressing directly over the patient's protective clothing. Also, do not attempt to decontaminate skin where blisters have formed. The fluid-filled blisters are keeping the underlying skin clean, which prevents infection.

Laser burns: Remove the laser burn casualty from the laser source. Be careful not to enter the beam yourself, or you too may become a casualty.

Never look directly at the beam source, and if possible wear appropriate eye protection.

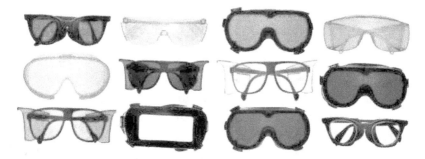

Appropriate eye protection for safety

Thermal burns: Remove the victim from the heat source and immediately provide first aid. If the victim's clothes are burning, have them stop, drop, and roll, or put out the fire with water, a fire hydrant, or a smothering blanket.

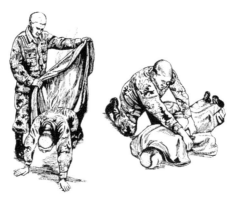

CATEGORIES OF BURNS

Regardless of their cause, burns are divided into three categories: first, second, and third degree. The degree of the burn is determined by the depth of the damage to the skin. The skin is the body's greatest defense against infection. Burns damage and compromise the skin, which can lead to not only infection, but also dehydration and possibly even hypothermia. The main goals in treating a burn are to stop the burning process, prevent shock, prevent infection, and ease pain. By determining the degree of burn, you can determine the type of care needed. The *U.S. Air Force Self Aid and Buddy Instructor Handbook* explains how to determine the type of the burn.

FIRST DEGREE BURNS

First degree burns are superficial and typically cause redness and pain to the outer layer of skin (epidermis). They usually heal with minimal treatment.

Signs and Symptoms

+ Redness of the skin

+ Swelling

+ Pain

Treatment

+ Cool the burned area with running water or a cold compress.

+ Apply topical burn ointment.

+ Cover and protect the burned area with a sterile gauze bandage.

+ Administer over-the-counter pain medication.

SECOND DEGREE BURNS

Second degree burns are slightly deeper into the second layer of skin (dermis) and cause significant pain and blistering. They may require advanced medical care if and when it becomes available.

Signs and Symptoms

+ Skin is deep red and splotchy

+ Significant pain and swelling

+ Blisters typically develop

Treatment

+ If the burn is small (less than 3 inches in diameter) and not located on the face, groin, hands, feet, or a major joint, treat as a first degree burn.

+ If the burn covers a large surface area or is located on one of the above-mentioned critical areas, treat as a third degree burn.

THIRD DEGREE BURNS

Third degree burns (also referred to as full-thickness burns) are the most serious burns, causing damage into the subcutaneous layers of skin and posing a significant health risk. Receiving advanced care can be critical in the case of a third degree burn. The skin can be black and charred or possibly dry and white.

Signs and Symptoms

+ Dry and leathery skin

+ Skin may be black, white, brown, or yellow

+ Swelling

+ Pain may be absent due to destroyed nerve endings

Treatment

+ Clean the wound with sterile water and remove loose debris.

+ Treat for shock.

+ Do not remove burned clothing stuck to the wound.

+ Cover the wound with loose sterile cloth.

+ If possible, elevate the wound.

+ If burns are to the face, check for breathing complications.

+ DO NOT apply ointment, cream, ice, fluffy wound dressing, or medications to the wound.

Avoid household burn remedies such as applying butter, pouring alcohol or milk, and placing cold meat on the wound. Only use medical ointments or aloe vera on first or second degree burns, but do not use ANY ointment on third degree burns.

CHAPTER 7
HEAT-RELATED EMERGENCIES

Heat emergencies may be the result of exposure to high ambient temperatures, not wearing proper clothing, or being inside warm places with little ventilation. They mostly occur during summer, but spring and fall are not free from the threat of heat. Exposure to elevated temperatures and sunlight place people at risk, and unless skin protection and hydration issues are addressed, the body cannot function normally, and its ability to regulate temperature becomes compromised. The nervous system regulates body temperature. As internal temperatures elevate, the body has a mechanism called thermoregulation in place to recognize the change and make adjustments. Sweating and changes in blood flow are the most common methods the body uses to cool itself. It is when those processes are not enough to cool the body that the internal temperature can become dangerous.

In the warm summer months, I respond to calls for heat-related emergencies, and the vast majority of the time it's due to someone working out in the heat. During the peak of summer, people are often aware of the dangers of high heat and take precautions against it. But during a typical warm weather day, people will let their guard down and go to work at their job or in their yard and neglect the early signs and symptoms of dehydration or more severe heat-related issues.

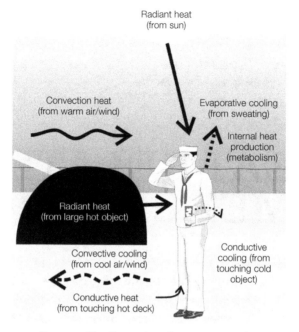

Sources of heating and cooling energy transfer

Heat exposure issues also become a problem in post-disaster situations when people are giving their all to help out whenever and wherever they can without ensuring their own well-being first. The 2010 earthquake in Haiti that took a reported 200,000 lives is a sad example of a disaster that occurred in high-humidity and high-heat conditions. The rescue workers and volunteers worked tirelessly to pull victims from the rubble while succumbing to their own heat-related medical issues. Even absent a typical natural disaster, excessive heat can become its own emergency. For example, in July 1995, the city of Chicago saw over 700 heat-related deaths.

Heat-related illnesses also occur often in wilderness situations. Whether it is a hiking excursion, camping trip, or a survival scenario, it is common for people to be ill-prepared for high ambient temperatures and the amount of water needed for a body that is actively working. Regardless of what has occurred to put someone in a hot and strenuous environment, specific attention should be paid to keeping the body cool, rested, and hydrated.

In a desert survival and evasion situation, it's unlikely that you will have a medic or medical supplies with you to treat heat injuries. Therefore, the *US Army Survival Manual* recommends the following precautions: Take extra care to avoid heat injuries; rest during the day; and work during the cool evenings and nights. Use a buddy system to watch for heat injury, and observe the following guidelines:

+ Make sure you tell someone where you're going and when you'll return.

+ Watch for signs of heat injury. If someone complains of tiredness or wanders away from the group, he may be a heat casualty.

+ Drink water at least once an hour.

+ Get in the shade when resting; do not lie directly on the ground.

+ Do not take off your shirt to work during the day.

+ Check the color of your urine. A light color means you are drinking enough water; a dark color means you need to drink more.

+ Wear protective lip balm with SPF protection.

One important part of preventing heat-related illnesses often left out of survival manuals is the simple use of sunscreen. Applying sunscreen at regular intervals will protect your skin from burns and your body from illnesses associated with sunburns, such as chills, fever, and nausea. Sunscreens are rated with a sun protection factor (SPF). A minimum of SPF 30 should be used. Ultraviolet B (UVB) rays are the cause of sunburn. SPF 15 blocks about 94 percent of UVB rays, SPF 30 blocks about 97 percent, and SPF 45 blocks about 98 percent. Any SPF rating above that is only marginally better, if at all. Regardless of the SPF rating you use, you should reapply often. The protection rating does not mean it will protect longer. Apply early and often to prevent ultraviolet injuries to your skin.

TYPES OF HEAT-RELATED ILLNESSES

There are four main heat-related issues: dehydration, heat cramps, heat exhaustion, and heatstroke. Heat cramps and heat exhaustion are mild, easily treatable heat-related illnesses. When identified early, dehydration is a mild, easily treatable condition, but if left uncorrected, it can become extremely dangerous. Heatstroke is a later-stage illness that is far more serious. Early recognition of the signs and symptoms is extremely important.

DEHYDRATION

Since the human body is primarily composed of water, it should be no surprise to find that fluids are vital to its normal functioning. Water maintains organ function, protects joints, and helps maintain body temperature. It doesn't take much to feel the effects of dehydration. In fact, some experts say that simply sleeping at night dehydrates the body and you should drink a glass of water to start the day. Obviously, that would be low-grade dehydration, but more severe dehydration occurs when you sweat excessively and are unable to replenish your body's water levels.

Signs and Symptoms

+ Decreased urine output and brighter yellow color

+ Headache

+ Dry mouth

+ Dry eyes

+ Dry skin

+ Light-headedness

+ Nausea

+ Heart palpitations

Treatment

+ Drink fluids. Water or sports drinks containing electrolytes will be your best options. You should avoid carbonated beverages, energy drinks, alcohol, and coffee. They can worsen dehydration and its effects.

+ If symptoms persist, seek medical treatment as soon as possible. Until advanced care is available, continue to provide fluids and keep the patient comfortable.

HEAT CRAMPS

Heat cramps are muscle cramps that occur most often in the arms, legs, or abdomen. They frequently occur in athletes who exert themselves and don't ingest enough fluids. According to the *US Army Survival Manual*, the loss of salt due to excessive sweating causes heat cramps. Symptoms are moderate to severe muscle cramps in the legs, arms, or abdomen. These symptoms may start as a mild muscular discomfort. If you experience muscle cramps, you should stop all activity, get in the shade, and drink water. If you fail to recognize the early symptoms and continue your physical activity, you'll have severe muscle cramps and pain, and you are at a greater risk for heat exhaustion or heatstroke.

Signs and Symptoms

+ Sweating

+ Muscular cramps or pain, typically in the abdomen, arms, or legs

Treatment

+ Stop all activity and sit quietly in a cool place.

+ Drink water or a sports beverage containing electrolytes.

+ Do not return to strenuous activity for a few hours after the cramps subside because further exertion may lead to heat exhaustion or heatstroke.

+ Seek medical attention for heat cramps if they do not subside in one hour. If advanced medical treatment is not available, continue to provide liquids for the patient and ensure they are as comfortable as possible until transport is an option.

HEAT EXHAUSTION

A large loss of body water and salt causes heat exhaustion. The body's average normal functioning temperature is 98.6°F (37°C). When it becomes overheated and dehydrated, the internal temperature can increase to a dangerous level. Typically, heat exhaustion occurs when someone exercises strenuously or overexerts themselves in hot or humid weather without taking the proper precautions to rest and hydrate. If caught and treated early enough, heat exhaustion is treatable and easily reversed. If allowed to progress untreated, it becomes a very dangerous scenario for the patient.

Signs and Symptoms

+ Heavy sweating

+ Paleness

+ Muscle cramps

+ Tiredness

+ Weakness

+ Dizziness

+ Headache

+ Nausea/vomiting

+ Fainting

Treatment

+ Drink cool, nonalcoholic beverages.

+ Rest.

+ Take a cool shower, bath, or sponge bath.

+ Seek an air-conditioned environment.

+ Wear lightweight clothing.

HEATSTROKE

Heatstroke is a condition that can be fatal if not recognized and treated immediately. In the *Manual of Naval Preventive Medicine*, it states in bold print that heatstroke is a medical emergency. People are often familiar with the term "hypothermia"—meaning a dangerously low body temperature—in cold-weather situations, but the opposite of that occurs in warm weather. The body goes into an elevated temperature or hyperthermic state. It doesn't take much internal temperature elevation to become dangerous. In fact, anything above normal body temperature is cause for concern and treatment. When someone is showing signs and symptoms of heatstroke, immediate measures should be taken.

Signs and Symptoms

+ An extremely high body temperature, above 103°F (39.4°C)

+ Red, hot, and dry skin (no sweating)

+ Rapid, strong pulse

+ Throbbing headache

+ Dizziness

+ Nausea

+ Confusion

+ Unconsciousness

Treatment

+ Get the victim to a shady area.

+ Cool the victim rapidly, using whatever methods you can. For example, immerse the victim in a tub of cool water; place the person in a cool shower; spray the victim with cool water from a garden hose; sponge them with cool water; or, if the humidity is low, wrap the victim in a cool, wet sheet, and fan him or her vigorously.

+ Monitor body temperature and continue cooling efforts until the body temperature drops to 101 to 102°F (38 to 39°C).

+ Do not give the victim alcohol to drink.

+ If emergency medical personnel are delayed, call the hospital emergency room for further instructions, if that is an option.

+ Get the patient advanced medical care as soon as possible. Until that is available, continue to take measures to lower the patient's core temperature and monitor their condition.

CHAPTER 8

COLD-RELATED EMERGENCIES

One of the most difficult survival situations is a cold-weather scenario. Remember, cold weather is an adversary that can be as dangerous as an enemy soldier. Every time you venture into the cold, you are pitting yourself against the elements. With a little knowledge of the environment, proper plans, and appropriate equipment, you can overcome the elements. As you remove one or more of these factors, survival becomes increasingly difficult. Remember, winter weather is highly variable. Prepare yourself to adapt to blizzard conditions even during sunny and clear weather. Cold is a far greater threat to survival than it appears. It decreases your ability to think and weakens your will to do anything except to get warm. Cold is an insidious enemy; as it numbs the mind and body, it subdues the will to survive. Cold makes it very easy to forget your ultimate goal—to survive.

—US Army Survival Manual

Troops participating in military deployments often encounter cold-temperature stress that requires management for them to successfully accomplish their mission. Excessive cold stress degrades physical performance capabilities, significantly impacts morale, and eventually leads to casualties. Cold stress environments include not only exposure to extremely low temperatures (for example, Arctic regions), but also cold–wet exposures (for example, rain, immersion in water) in warmer ambient temperatures.

Cold injuries are surprisingly possible in nearly any environment. Even in a desert, blistering daytime temperatures plummet to dangerous lows at night. However, cold-related emergencies are most likely to occur when conditions are moderately cold and accompanied by moisture or wind. The body loses its ability to maintain a safe internal temperature. The cold becomes problematic when the body's core temperature drops below the normal 98.6°F (37°C). If it continues to drop, people are at risk of hypothermia. Hypothermia occurs when the body's temperature continues to drop below what it requires for normal function, which by definition is 95°F (35°C).

The military technical bulletin *Prevention and Management of Cold-Weather Injuries* states that cold-induced injuries usually begin as a localized peripheral insult to the extremities and progress (or regress) to a cooling of the entire body. Since your limbs and head have less protective body tissue than your torso, their temperatures vary and may not reach core temperature. Your body has a control system that lets it react to temperature extremes to maintain a balance. There are three main factors that affect this temperature balance: heat production, heat loss, and evaporation.

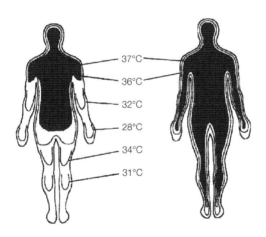

Effects of cold (left) and heat (right)

The difference between the body's core temperature and the environment's temperature governs the heat production rate. Obviously, as external temperatures decrease, your body will take strides to combat the cooling process. One of those mechanisms is the act of involuntary movement— shivering. Shivering causes the body to generate heat, but it also causes fatigue that, in turn, leads to a drop in body temperature. Shivering is an obvious external sign that the body's internal temperature is dropping, and action should be taken to begin warming it.

Air movement around your body affects heat loss. It has been calculated that a naked man exposed to still air at or around −32°F (0°C) can maintain a heat balance if he shivers as hard as he can. However, he can't shiver forever. It has also been calculated that a man at rest wearing the maximum arctic clothing in a cold environment can keep his internal heat balance in temperatures well below freezing. To withstand extreme cold conditions for any length of time, however, he will have to become active or shiver.

The severity of the injury depends on several factors, such as duration of exposure, temperature, if protective clothing was worn, and overall general health of the victim. The best way to handle cold-weather emergencies is to deal with them before they occur. Cold injuries can usually be prevented. Those offering to render aid need to be aware of the conditions and be prepared as well. The coldest my hands have ever been was out in bitter cold temperatures, wearing nitrile gloves, and rendering aid to victims of a car crash. My fingers were wrapped in protective gloves that offer zero thermal protection and deny them the benefit of body heat from adjacent fingers. In mere minutes, my fingers were numb and painful. Well-disciplined and well-prepared people can be protected even in the most adverse circumstances. They must know the hazards of cold-weather exposure and the importance of exercise, care of the feet and hands, and the use of protective clothing.

TYPES OF COLD-WEATHER INJURIES

Cold-weather injuries are basically broken down into two categories: frostbite and hypothermia.

FROSTBITE

Frostbite is the result of frozen tissue. Light frostbite involves only the skin, which takes on a dull, whitish pallor. Deep frostbite extends below the skin, and the tissue becomes solid and immovable. Your feet, hands, and exposed facial areas are particularly vulnerable to frostbite. The best frostbite prevention, when you're with others, is to use the buddy system.

Check your buddy's face often, and make sure that they check yours. If you're alone, periodically cover your nose and lower part of your face with your gloved hand. The following pointers will aid you in keeping warm and preventing frostbite when it's extremely cold or when you have less than adequate clothing:

+ **Face**: Maintain circulation by twitching and wrinkling the skin on your face, making faces. Warm with your hands.

+ **Ears**: Wiggle and move your ears. Warm with your hands.

+ **Hands**: Move your hands inside your gloves. Warm by placing your hands close to your body, or in the warmest places of your body, the armpits and the groin.

+ **Feet**: Move your feet and wiggle your toes inside your boots.

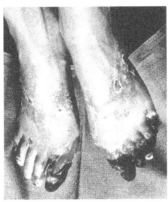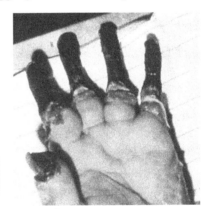

Examples of frostbite

Signs and Symptoms

+ Feeling numbness, burning, tingling, or itching

+ Skin turning red, white, or blueish, or having a yellow tint

+ Waxy-looking skin

+ Blisters

Treatment

+ Move the patient out of the cold and into a warm place.

+ Remove wet clothing and jewelry.

+ Give the patient warm, nonalcoholic drinks.

+ Apply a dry, sterile bandage over the affected area to protect it. Do not rub the skin.

+ Body heat can be used to passively warm an affected area. The warmest areas of the body are the groin and the armpits, so if possible, put the frostbitten area near those areas.

+ If a small part of the body is affected, such as a hand or foot, you can soak the area in warm (*not* hot) water.

+ Pain medication such as ibuprofen can be taken as long as the patient can tolerate it. The rewarming process can be painful.

+ DO NOT actively warm the body, because the skin is numb and so is at risk of burning. (For example: Laying the victim next to a campfire is dangerous).

+ DO NOT walk if toes or feet have been frostbitten. Further damage may occur.

+ DO NOT warm someone if there is a chance of refreezing.

A loss of feeling in your hands and feet is a sign of frostbite. If you have lost feeling for only a short time, the frostbite is probably light. Otherwise, assume the frostbite is deep. To rewarm a light frostbite, use your hands or mittens to warm your face and ears. Place your hands under your armpits. Place your feet next to your buddy's stomach. A deep frostbite injury, if thawed and refrozen, will cause more damage than a non–medically trained person can handle. Transport the person to advanced care as soon as possible.

HYPOTHERMIA

Hypothermia is the lowering of the body temperature at a rate faster than the body can produce heat. Causes of hypothermia may be general exposure or the sudden wetting of the body by falling into a lake or by being sprayed with a liquid.

Progressive Symptoms

1. The initial symptom is shivering. This shivering may progress to the point where it is uncontrollable and interferes with an individual's ability to care for themselves. According to the military technical bulletin *Prevention and Management of Cold-Weather Injuries*, this begins when the body's core temperature falls to about 96°F (35.5°C).

2. When the core temperature reaches 95 to 90°F (35 to 32°C), sluggish thinking, irrational reasoning, and a false feeling of warmth may occur.

3. Core temperatures of 90 to 86°F (32 to 30°C) and below result in muscle rigidity, unconsciousness, and barely detectable signs of life.

4. If the victim's core temperature falls below 77°F (25°C), death is almost certain.

Treatment

1. First and foremost, move the victim into a warm environment.

2. If the victim's clothes are wet, remove them.

3. Begin active rewarming by placing the victim under loose, dry layers. Gently rub the skin *only* if no signs of frostbite exist. If there are signs of frostbite, do not rub the skin, or skin and tissue damage can occur.

4. Give ibuprofen. The re-warming process can be painful.

5. Consider treating with aloe vera. Aloe can be effective for treating frostbite because it has been proven to increase blood flow to affected areas. The increased blood flow allows the restricted vessels the opportunity to expand and repair, while simultaneously reducing pain, redness, swelling, and inflammation.

6. Drink warm beverages. Some literature advises against drinking fluids of any kind in cold-weather injury scenarios, but if the patient can maintain their own airway, there is a psychological benefit to allowing them to sip a warm beverage. Alcohol should be avoided. It is counterproductive to the body's natural processes. Alcohol increases blood flow to the skin, giving the person the feeling of warmth, when actually the body's core temperature could be continuing to decrease.

7. If hypothermia is suspected (shivering, confusion, memory loss), do not immerse the victim in warm water, as it can cause heart arrhythmia. Instead, warm the person with layers of warm, dry blankets, and, if possible, use the body heat of another person.

CHAPTER 9
ALLERGIC REACTIONS

Allergic reactions are extremely common, and when the reaction is minor, there may be no intervention needed at all. You may have even experienced one and not known it. It could be a food allergy that causes a small rash or a little bit of scratchiness in your throat. As with most things, the human body does an amazing job of taking care of itself. The adverse reaction occurs when the body identifies something as a threat. It begins to fight the substance, which is often harmless, such as medication, pollen, dust mites, food, and so on. The result can be minor issues (rash, itchy eyes, runny nose) or a more severe reaction (difficulty breathing or nausea). Allergic reactions are not necessarily a medical emergency. However, a severe reaction, called anaphylaxis, *is*.

To understand the treatment of allergic reactions, you should understand what's happening, beginning with knowing and understanding some of the terms associated with the allergic reactions.

Simply put, an *allergen* is a substance that the body's immune system recognizes as a threat, triggering an allergic reaction. They can be found in food, drinks, perfumes, metals, the environment, or really anywhere. A person can be allergic to just about anything, but most times the allergen is harmless. Even a sneeze is a reaction to an allergen. It is with more severe sensitivities that significant medical issues can arise.

Histamine is a chemical found in some cells of the body that causes many of the symptoms associated with allergic reactions. A runny nose, sneezing, and itchy eyes are all symptoms of a response to histamine. When someone is allergic to something in particular, the body believes that substance is actually harmful. In an attempt to protect itself, the body prompts cells to release histamine into the bloodstream, which, in turn, will engage an attempt to flush the "harmful" substance. That is why you'll see medication advertised as an "antihistamine," which will reduce or block histamines, offering relief of the symptoms.

COMMON TYPES OF ALLERGIES

Airborne allergies: Chances are, either you or someone you know is affected by airborne allergies. Pollen, dust, mold, and so on are examples of airborne allergies. People affected by airborne allergies are all too familiar with having a runny nose, itchy/watery eyes, and sinus inflammation due to allergens. Approximately one-third of the population of developed countries are affected. When an allergen comes in contact with the mucous membranes lining the inside of the nose, a chain reaction occurs that leads the cells in these tissues to release histamine. These powerful chemicals contract the cells that line blood vessels inside the nose. This allows fluids to escape, which causes the nasal passages to swell, resulting in nasal congestion. Common antihistamine medications, such as Allegra, Claritin, and Benadryl, are typically used to treat the reaction. They suppress the body's reaction and reduce the amount of congestion that occurs with the release of histamine.

Drug allergies: Drug allergies are also very common. During any kind of medical assessment, one of the questions that health-care professionals will ask is if you are allergic to any medications. They do this because drug allergies are common, and health-care workers don't want to accidentally make you worse by giving you a medication that you are allergic to. The most common drug allergies are antibiotic (such as penicillin and sulfa drugs) and nonsteroidal anti-inflammatory drugs such as aspirin. Like other allergic reactions, a hypersensitivity to medications can present as a mild irritation or can be a life-threatening condition that should be treated by medical professionals as soon as possible.

Food allergies: In 2004, Congress passed the Food Allergen Labeling and Consumer Protection Act so that people could more easily identify the most common allergens contained in foods. That act identified the eight most common food ingredients that cause allergic reactions: crustaceans, eggs, milk, fish, nuts, peanuts, soybeans, and wheat. According to the Centers for Disease Control (CDC), over 50 million Americans have a food allergy of some kind. The majority of food-related allergic reactions occur within two hours of ingestion, while more rare cases can take up to six hours to show signs or symptoms.

Insect allergies: If you are not allergic to bee stings, you probably know someone who is. Honeybees, bumblebees, yellow jackets, yellow hornets, and paper wasps are responsible for the majority of stings that create a reaction in the body. An insect bite or sting can cause great pain, allergic reaction, inflammation, and infection. If not treated correctly, some bites/stings may cause serious illness or even death. When an allergic reaction is not involved, first aid is a simple process (see Chapter 1). In any case, medical personnel should examine the casualty as soon as possible. It is important to properly identify the spider, bee, or creature that caused the bite/sting, especially in cases of allergic reaction.

Skin allergies: Most skin contact allergy cases are mild and come courtesy of plants such as poison ivy, poison oak, and poison sumac. However, other common sources do exist, such as skin reactions to certain metals, perfumes, and latex. Unless someone has a severe sensitivity, most skin allergies cause only redness and itchiness and are easily treatable.

SIGNS AND SYMPTOMS

There is no way to predict how severe a reaction will become or if advanced medical care will be needed. A severe allergic reaction, called anaphylaxis, can quickly become deadly. Common anaphylactic reactions can include any or all of the following: swelling, hives, decreased blood pressure, and airway restriction. If an anaphylactic reaction occurs, call 911 immediately (if possible). If advanced medical care is not available, follow treatment steps until help arrives. Signs and symptoms can be any or all of the following:

Mild Symptoms:

+ Rash

+ Localized itching

+ Itchy and watery eyes

+ Congestion

Moderate Symptoms:

+ Widespread itching

+ Difficulty breathing

Severe Symptoms:

+ Difficulty swallowing

+ Increased difficulty breathing

+ Cramps

+ Abdominal pain

+ Vomiting

+ Diarrhea

+ Altered mental status

+ Dizziness

TREATMENT

Treating minor symptoms of an allergic reaction involves taking over-the-counter medication. Antihistamines, decongestants, nasal sprays, and eyedrops are just a few of the options that offer relief of the minor symptoms of an allergic reaction. Minor to moderate allergic reactions cause discomfort and cosmetic issues, but often little beyond that. Because there is no way of predicting how severe a reaction will be, the patient should be watched closely for worsening conditions and transported to a medical facility when necessary and possible.

Many times people with a known severe allergy will carry the blood-pressure raising hormone epinephrine in the form of an EpiPen. An EpiPen is a self-administered, measured medication that can be injected in the case of an anaphylactic reaction. That person should be familiar with it and can usually tell you how to administer it.

Do not administer epinephrine until you've ensured the five "rights":

1. **Right person**: The epinephrine is prescribed to the person in need.

2. **Right medication**: The medication you are going to help administer is epinephrine.

3. **Right dose**: The correct dose is one full injection of epinephrine—the entire contents of one EpiPen.

4. **Right route**: You are injecting the dose in the correct way and at the correct place.

5. **Right time**: You are injecting the dose when someone is showing signs and symptoms of a life-threatening allergic reaction.

EpiPen administration:

1. Identify that an anaphylactic reaction is taking place.

2. Call 911 if it's an option. If not, follow treatment steps until help arrives.

3. Check the person for an emergency medical ID necklace or bracelet that contains critical medical information.

4. Ensure the five "rights."

5. Remove the safety cap.

6. Hold the EpiPen firmly in your fist without placing your thumb over the end.

7. Press firmly into the muscular part of the patient's thigh and hold; 10 seconds should be more than enough.

8. Remove the EpiPen.

9. Massage injection site for 10 seconds.

10. Be prepared for the patient to feel anxious, panicked, or even shaky—all common reactions to epinephrine.

11. Transport the patient to an advanced medical care facility as soon as possible. If there is no EpiPen available, you should take steps to remove the patient from whatever caused the allergic reaction. Monitor their ABCs and give supportive care, such as CPR, if needed. In a disaster situation, immediate 911 response is not likely, so follow these treatment steps until help arrives.

CHAPTER 10

✚
CHAPTER 10
BITES AND STINGS

There are likely few people who have not received an insect bite or sting from one creature or another. You don't have to be out in nature to be a victim—nature finds its way to you. Insects such as bees, wasps, fleas, and mosquitoes, as well as arachnids such as spiders, ticks, and scorpions, have a tendency to sting or bite when provoked or distressed. Occasionally, the victim isn't even aware that it has occurred, but more often than not, the bite or sting is initially painful followed by discomfort and possibly an allergic reaction.

Less common, but possibly more frightening, is a snakebite. In the United States there are over 20 species of venomous snakes. Hawaii and Alaska are the only states free from a known species of venomous snake. The majority of snakebites are from more common and less lethal varieties. Localized pain and redness occur in over 90 percent of snakebites, but, particularly in North America, such bites are rarely fatal. The danger, though, is very real and should be taken seriously. The outcome will depend on the type of snake, the location of the bite, the amount of venom introduced by the fangs, and the general health of the victim.

There are also an alarming number of reported human bites every year, ranking third among bite cases seen in emergency departments, behind bites from dogs and cats. As odd as it sounds, human bites can be extremely dangerous—not so much from the bite itself, but from the bacteria introduced into the victim's body. Human, dog, and cat bites are all treated very similarly in the field. Knowledge and prompt application of first aid measures can lessen the severity of injuries from bites and stings and keep the patient from becoming a serious casualty.

Any type of bite or sting can be harmless on one end of the spectrum and lethal on the other. The danger lies in the unknown. What type of creature inflicted the bite or sting? Is it poisonous? If so, how much venom was injected into the body? Is the creature diseased? What will be the human body's reaction to it? Because you may not know answers to any number of those questions, you should immediately treat the patient, obtain as much information about who or what inflicted the bite/sting, and transport them to a medical facility.

HUMAN/ANIMAL BITES

When people discuss and prepare to treat for bites, human bites are rarely considered. Statistically, a human bite is rarer than an animal bite, but it's a frequent enough occurrence that you should be prepared to treat the injury just as you would an animal bite. A common scenario is a child biting another child, but it also happens between adults, often as an assault. Keep in mind that if one person throws a punch at another person and hits them in the mouth, if the person who threw the punch receives a cut to the hand, that is still considered a human bite and should be treated as such.

Bites from humans and other animals, such as dogs, cats, bats, raccoons, and rats, can cause severe bruises and tears or lacerations of tissue. In addition to damaging tissue, bites also always present the possibility of infection. Awareness of the potential sources of injuries can reduce or eliminate the likelihood of infection.

Human bites that break the skin may become seriously infected since the mouth is heavily contaminated with bacteria. The infection is often far worse than the damage done to the skin and blood loss from the bite itself.

Animal bites can result in both infection and disease. Tetanus, rabies, and various types of fevers can follow an untreated animal bite. Because of these possible complications, the animal causing the bite should, if possible, be captured or killed (without damaging its head) so that it can be tested for disease.

SIGNS AND SYMPTOMS

An infected bite, whether it comes from a human or an animal, can have any or all of the following symptoms:

+ Swelling around the area of the bite

+ Heat around the site of the bite

+ Pus discharge

+ Pain or tenderness around the area of the bite

+ Chills

+ Fever

TREATMENT

+ Cleanse the wound thoroughly with soap, flush it well with water, and cover it with a sterile dressing.

+ Immobilize the injured arm or leg, if appropriate.

+ Transport the casualty immediately to a medical facility.

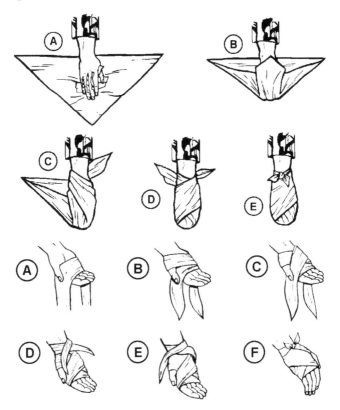

Ways to bandage a bitten hand

INSECT BITES

Insects can be problematic in any type of environment, even when you're just relaxing at home. The majority of issues, though, occur outside—in open fields and forests, near streams and ponds, in backyards and on playgrounds. Most stings and insect bites cause little more than minor irritation and redness. The best way to avoid the complications of insect bites and stings is to keep immunizations (including booster shots) up to date, avoid insect-infested areas, use netting and insect repellent, and wear all clothing properly. If you get bitten or stung, do not scratch the bite or sting, or it might become infected. Inspect your body at least once a day to ensure there are no insects attached to you, particularly if you have spent any time in grassy or wooded areas.

The bite or sting itself can be only a small part of a bigger issue. Insects have been known to carry a variety of easily transmittable diseases.

TICKS, MOSQUITOES, FLIES, FLEAS, AND LICE

Ticks: Ticks are extremely common unwelcome passengers on your body any time you travel through grassy or wooded areas. They can carry and transmit diseases, such as Lyme disease and Rocky Mountain spotted fever, common in many parts of the United States. When spending time in the wilderness,

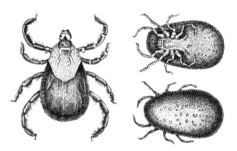

Types of ticks: hard (left) and soft (right)

check your body frequently for ticks. Many experts believe it can take hours for a tick to transmit a disease, so locating them quickly and removing them is a must. Again, repellent will be your best bet to keep them away from you, but you can also try tucking your pants into your socks to reduce the chances of one hitching a ride. Military manuals recommend that if you find ticks attached to your body, you should cover them with a substance, such as Vaseline, heavy oil, or tree sap, that will cut off their air supply. Without air, the tick releases its hold, and you can remove it. Take care to remove the whole tick. Use tweezers if you have them. Grasp the tick where the mouth parts are attached to the skin. Do not squeeze the tick's body. Wash your hands after touching the tick. Clean the wound daily until healed.

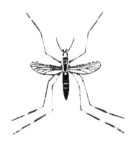

Mosquitoes: These bugs are famous for transmitting disease, as they tap into blood sources wherever they can find them. They may carry malaria, dengue, and many other diseases, and are best avoided with repellent and by covering as much of your skin as possible, using fine netting to cover your face and head.

Flies: Flies can spread disease from contact with infectious sources. They are causes of sleeping sickness, typhoid, cholera, and dysentery.

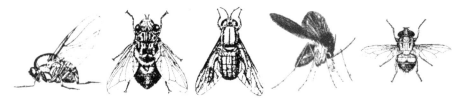

Types of flies: (from left to right) black flies, bot flies, deer flies, sand flies, tumbu flies

Fleas: Fleas can transmit plague.

Lice: Lice can transmit typhus and relapsing fever.

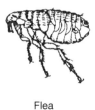
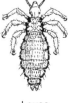

Flea   Louse

Signs and Symptoms

+ Swelling

+ Itching

+ Rash or redness of the affected area

+ Pain in the affected area

Treatment

It is impossible to list the treatments of all the different types of bites and stings. *The vast majority of the population should treat bites and stings topically and seek medical attention if signs and symptoms worsen.*

If you are medically trained, the *US Army Survival Manual* recommends treating bites and stings as follows:

+ If antibiotics are available, become familiar with them before deployment for your use.

+ Predeployment immunizations can prevent most of the common diseases carried by mosquitoes and some carried by flies.

+ The common fly-borne diseases are usually treatable with penicillin or erythromycin.

+ Most tick-, flea-, louse-, and mite-borne diseases are treatable with tetracycline.

Most antibiotics come in 250 mg or 500 mg tablets. If you cannot remember the exact dose rate to treat a disease, two tablets, four times a day for 10 to 14 days will usually kill any bacteria.

BEE AND WASP STINGS

If stung by a bee, immediately remove the stinger and venom sac, if attached, by scraping with a fingernail or a knife blade. Do not squeeze or grasp the stinger or venom sac, as squeezing will force more venom into the wound. Wash the sting site thoroughly with soap and water to lessen the chance of a secondary infection. If you know or suspect that you are allergic to insect stings, always carry an insect sting kit with you. The *US Army Survival Manual* states, "Even more victims die [each year] from allergic reactions to bee stings" than from venomous snakes or large dangerous animals.

Signs and Symptoms of a Severe Allergic Reaction

+ Swelling around the lips, eyes, tongue, or throat

+ Itching

+ Rash or hives

+ Wheezing

+ Dizziness

+ Stomach cramps

+ Difficulty breathing

+ Difficulty swallowing

Treatment

Relieve the itching and discomfort caused by insect bites by applying:

+ Cold compresses

+ A cooling paste of mud and ashes

+ Sap from dandelions

+ Coconut meat

+ Crushed cloves of garlic

+ A slice of raw onion

SPIDERS AND SCORPIONS

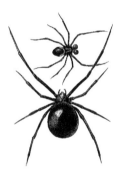

Black widow spider: male (top) and female (bottom)

Black widow spider: The black widow spider is identified by a red hourglass on its abdomen. Only the female bites, and it has a neurotoxic venom. The initial pain is not terrible, but severe local pain rapidly develops. The pain gradually spreads over the entire body and settles in the abdomen and legs. Abdominal cramps and progressive nausea, vomiting, and a rash may occur, as may weakness, tremors, sweating, and salivation. Anaphylactic reactions can occur. Symptoms begin to regress after several hours and are usually gone in a few days.

Signs and Symptoms

+ Severe pain, starting around the bite and spreading over the entire body, settling in the abdomen and legs

+ Abdominal cramps

+ Nausea/vomiting

+ Rash

+ Weakness

+ Tremors

+ Sweating

+ Salivation

+ Anaphylactic reactions (see page 50)

Treatment

If someone is bitten by a black widow, the *US Army Survival Manual* recommends that you:

+ Treat the patient for shock.

+ Be ready to perform CPR.

+ Clean and dress the bite area to reduce the risk of infection.

+ Administer an antivenin if it is available and you are trained to do so.

Funnel-web spider: The funnel-web spider is a large brown or gray spider common in Australia, though it can also be found throughout North America. There are actually several kinds of funnel-web spiders; some are nonpoisonous and others, such as the Sydney funnel-web spider, are among the most venomous spiders in the world. Their presence is indicated by a unique, sheet-like web with a funnel leading downward toward a shelter. The most common funnel-web spiders found in North America have a lightly hairy and roundish carapace featuring two broad, dark-brownish bands running lengthwise and a parallel lighter middle band. Most funnel-web spiders encountered in North America are harmless to humans, though depending on the exact type of spider and the person receiving the bite, adverse reactions can occur.

Signs and Symptoms

+ Nausea

+ Difficulty breathing

+ Body fluid secretions such as saliva and tears

+ Heavy coughing

+ Joint pain

+ Muscle spasms

+ Sweating

+ Diarrhea

Treatment

+ Calm the patient.

+ Apply a bandage and put firm pressure over the bite.

+ Keep the wound site as still as possible and splint if necessary.

+ Remove clothing and jewelry that would be constricted by swelling

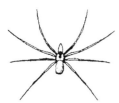

Brown recluse spider: The brown recluse spider is a small, light-brown spider identified by a dark brown violin-shaped marking on its back. The outstanding characteristic of the brown recluse bite is an ulcer that does not heal but persists for weeks or months. There is no pain or so little pain that some victims are not aware of the bite at first. Within a few hours, a painful red area with a mottled cyanotic center appears. Necrosis does not occur in all bites, but usually in three to four days, a star-shaped, firm area of deep purple discoloration appears at the bite site. The area turns dark and mummified in a week or two. The margins separate and the scab falls off, leaving an open ulcer. Secondary infection and regional swollen lymph glands usually become visible at this stage. In addition to the ulcer, there is often a systemic reaction that is serious and may lead to death. Reactions (fever, chills, joint pain, vomiting, and a generalized rash) occur chiefly in children or debilitated persons.

Signs and Symptoms

+ Reddened skin

+ Possible blister at the site of the bite

+ An open sore and breakdown of tissue at the site over the days following the bite

+ Pain

+ Fever

+ Chills

+ Generalized rash

+ Nausea/vomiting

Treatment

+ Calm the patient.

+ Apply a cool, wet towel to the site.

+ Use over-the-counter pain relief medication.

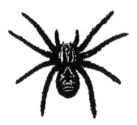

Tarantula: Tarantulas are large, hairy spiders found mainly in the tropics. Most do not inject venom, but some South American species do. They have large fangs. If you're bitten, pain and bleeding are certain, and infection is likely. Treat this type of bite as you would any open wound, and try to prevent infection. Tarantulas have a nasty reputation, but there are no records of a bite causing a human fatality. Though all tarantulas are venomous and some bites can cause significant pain and even hallucinations, the majority of tarantula bites feel similar to the sting of a wasp. If symptoms of poisoning appear, treat as for the bite of the black widow spider (see page 95).

Signs and Symptoms

+ Pain at the site of the bite

+ Difficulty breathing

+ Itching

+ Low blood pressure

+ Rapid heart rate

+ Swelling at the site, lips, throat, or eyes

Treatment

+ Wash the area with soap and water.

+ Place an ice pack over the site for 10 minutes and then off for 10 minutes, then repeat once more.

+ Apply topical cortisone or Benadryl (antihistamine) cream to reduce irritation.

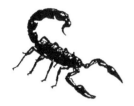 **Scorpion**: These distant cousins of spiders are all poisonous to some degree. The *US Marine Corps Summer Survival Course Handbook* warns that a scorpion sting could lead to very dangerous respiratory distress.

Signs and Symptoms

There are two different reactions to scorpion stings, depending on the species.

1. Severe local reaction only, affecting just the area of the bite.
This type of reaction includes the following symptoms:

+ Pain and swelling around the area of the sting

+ Prickly sensation around the mouth

+ Thick-feeling tongue

2. Severe systemic reaction, with little or no visible local reaction.
Local pain may be present. This type of reaction includes the following symptoms:

+ Respiratory difficulties

+ Thick-feeling tongue

+ Body spasms, drooling

+ Gastric distention

+ Double vision

+ Blindness

+ Involuntary rapid movement of the eyeballs

+ Involuntary urination and defecation

+ Heart failure

Death is rare, occurring mainly in children and adults with high blood pressure or illnesses. Treat scorpion stings as you would a black widow bite (see page 95).

MARINE STINGS AND BITES

With the exception of sharks, most marine animals will not deliberately attack. The most frequent injuries from marine animals are wounds by biting, stinging, or puncturing, most often in what they perceive as self-defense. Wounds inflicted by marine animals can be very painful, but are rarely fatal.

SHARKS, BARRACUDAS, AND ALLIGATORS

Wounds from these animals can involve major trauma as a result of bites and lacerations. Bites from large marine animals are potentially the most life-threatening of all injuries. Sharks, according to the *US Army Survival Manual*, can be especially aggressive, have an acute sense of smell, and sense abnormal vibrations in the water indicative of potential prey.

There usually isn't any doubt whether or not you've been bitten by one of these creatures. All have mouths full of flesh-tearing teeth powered by some of the strongest jaws on the planet. Mangled flesh and muscle accompanied by significant blood loss are the telltale signs of a shark, barracuda, or alligator bite. Immediate care is critical.

Treatment

+ Control bleeding.

+ Prevent shock.

+ Give basic life support.

+ Splint any injuries if necessary.

+ Seek medical aid as soon as possible. Until the patient can receive advanced care, ensure they are comfortable, and monitor them for changes.

TURTLES, MORAY EELS, AND CORALS

Though eels can be several feet of solid muscle, jaws, and teeth, and snapping turtles are relatives of alligators, these creatures normally inflict only minor wounds. Turtles and eels, when they do bite, often take small chunks of flesh with them the size of their mouth, leaving behind torn flesh and muscle. Even coral is relatively harmless, but the right species can be lethal. Be able to accurately identify the types of coral and potential dangers. Injuries from all these creatures should be treated immediately.

Treatment

+ Cleanse the wound(s) thoroughly.

+ Splint if necessary.

+ Seek advanced care as soon as possible.

JELLYFISH, PORTUGUESE MAN-OF-WAR, AND ANEMONES

These marine creatures, as well as others, inflict injury by means of stinging cells in their tentacles.

Symptoms

+ Burning pain, rash, and small hemorrhages where tentacles contacted skin

+ Shock

+ Muscular cramping

+ Nausea/vomiting

+ Respiratory distress

Treatment

+ Gently remove the clinging tentacles with a towel.

+ Wash or treat the area with diluted ammonia or alcohol, seasoned meat tenderizer, or talcum powder.

+ Keep the patient comfortable, and monitor them until advanced medical care can be obtained.

SPINY FISH, URCHINS, STINGRAYS, AND CONE SHELLS

These creatures inject their venom by puncturing the skin with their spines. Death as a result of these injuries is rare.

Signs and Symptoms

+ Swelling

+ Nausea

+ Vomiting

+ Generalized cramps

+ Diarrhea

+ Muscular paralysis

+ Shock

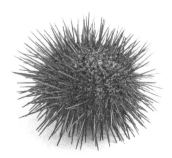

Sea urchin

Treatment

+ Soak the wounds in hot water (when available) for 30 to 60 minutes. This inactivates the heat-sensitive toxin.

+ Control bleeding as necessary.

SNAKEBITES

The chance of a snakebite in a survival situation is rather small if you're familiar with the various types of snakes and their habitats. Deaths from snakebites are rare. More than one-half of snakebite victims have little or no poisoning, and only about one-quarter develop serious systemic poisoning. However, it could happen, and you should know how to treat a snakebite. Failure to take preventive measures or to treat a snakebite properly can result in needless tragedy. A snakebite in a survival situation can be extremely painful and, beyond any medical issues, can greatly affect morale.

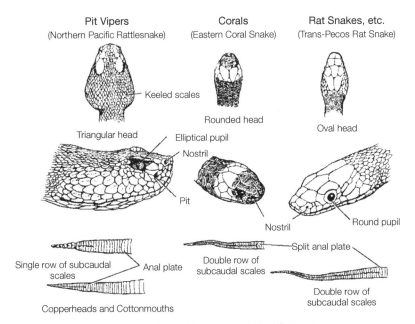

Pit Vipers	Corals	Rat Snakes, etc.
(Northern Pacific Rattlesnake)	(Eastern Coral Snake)	(Trans-Pecos Rat Snake)

Keeled scales

Rounded head

Oval head

Triangular head

Elliptical pupil

Nostril

Pit

Nostril

Round pupil

Single row of subcaudal scales

Anal plate

Split anal plate

Double row of subcaudal scales

Double row of subcaudal scales

Copperheads and Cottonmouths

Types of snakes and how to identify them

According to the *US Marine Corps Summer Survival Course Handbook*, the primary concern in the treatment of snakebites is to limit the amount of eventual tissue destruction around the bite area. A bite wound, regardless of the type of animal that inflicted it, can become infected from bacteria in the animal's mouth. With nonpoisonous as well as poisonous snakebites, this local infection is responsible for a large part of the residual damage that results. Snake venoms contain not only poisons that attack the victim's central nervous system (neurotoxins) and blood circulation (hemotoxins), but also digestive enzymes (cytotoxins) to aid in digesting their prey. These poisons can cause a very large area of tissue death, leaving a large, open wound. This condition could lead to the need for eventual amputation if not treated.

Shock and panic in a person bitten by a snake can also affect their recovery. Excitement, hysteria, and panic can speed up the circulation, causing the body to absorb the toxin quickly. Signs of shock occur within the first 30 minutes after the bite.

Before you start treating a snakebite, determine whether the snake was poisonous or nonpoisonous. *Nonpoisonous snakebites* will show rows of teeth. These bites should be treated like any other animal bite in order to reduce chances of infection. *Poisonous snakebites* may have rows of teeth showing, but will have one or more distinctive puncture marks caused by fang penetration.

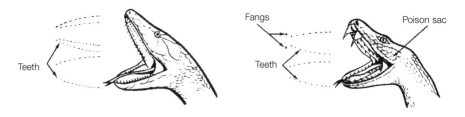

The difference between nonpoisonous (left) and poisonous (right) snakes and their bites

Signs and Symptoms of a Poisonous Snakebite

+ Fang puncture wounds

+ Pain at the site of the bite

+ Redness and swelling near the site of the bite within a few minutes or up to two hours later

+ Nausea

+ Vomiting

+ Dizziness

+ Blurred vision

+ Sweating

+ Numbness and tingling

+ Spontaneous bleeding from the nose and anus

+ Blood in the urine

+ Difficulty breathing

+ Paralysis

+ Weakness

+ Twitching

These signs and symptoms usually appear 90 minutes to two hours after the bite.

Treatment for a Poisonous Snakebite

If you determine that a poisonous snake bit an individual, immediately take the following steps:

+ Reassure the victim and keep them still.

+ Treat for shock and force fluids or give intravenous (IV) fluids if you're certified to do so and have the adequate supplies.

+ Remove watches, rings, bracelets, or other constricting items.

+ Clean the bite area.

+ Maintain an airway (especially if the bite is near the face or neck) and be prepared to administer CPR.

+ Use a constricting band between the wound and the heart.

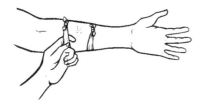

+ Immobilize the site.

+ Remove the poison as soon as possible by using a mechanical suction device or by squeezing.

DO NOT:

+ Give the victim alcoholic beverages or tobacco products.

+ Give morphine or other central nervous system (CNS) depressors.

+ Make any deep cuts at the bite site. Cutting opens capillaries that in turn open a direct route into the blood stream for venom and infection. (See "When Medical Help Is Over an Hour Away" on page 106.)

+ Put your hands on your face or rub your eyes, as venom may be on your hands. Venom may cause blindness.

+ Break open the large blisters that form around the bite site.

After caring for the victim as described, take the following actions to minimize local effects:

+ If infection appears, keep the wound open and clean.

+ Use heat after 24 to 48 hours to help prevent the spread of local infection. Heat also helps to draw out an infection.

+ Keep the wound covered with a dry, sterile dressing.

+ Have the victim drink large amounts of fluids until the infection is gone.

WHEN MEDICAL HELP IS OVER AN HOUR AWAY

If medical treatment is over one hour away, the US Army Survival Manual recommends an advanced technique if you have the proper training and certification.

1. Make an incision (no longer than 6 mm/¼ in and no deeper than 3 mm/⅛ in) over each puncture, cutting just deep enough to enlarge the fang opening, but only through the first or second layer of skin.

2. Place a suction cup over the bite so that you have a good vacuum seal.

3. Suction the bite site three to four times. (Use mouth suction *only as a last resort and only if you do not have open sores in your mouth.* Spit the envenomed blood out and rinse your mouth with water.) This method will draw out 25 to 30 percent of the venom.

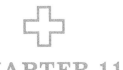

CHAPTER 11

COMMON MEDICAL EMERGENCIES

Every day, 911 dispatchers take calls from frantic people reporting medical emergencies. Fire trucks, police cars, and ambulances rush to the scenes to administer aid as quickly as possible. When they arrive, professionals with the latest training and up-to-date medical equipment begin treatment immediately. The responders' main goal is to stop a bad situation from getting worse and stabilize the patient or patients until they can be delivered to the emergency room. Whether or not a 911 response is an option, the most important thing you can do in a medical emergency is to quickly identify it.

For the purposes of this chapter, medical emergencies are considered episodes that occur inside the body that cannot be treated by standard first aid, such as chest pain and seizures. In the case of most medical incidents, there is little that can be done in the field beyond recognition and getting the patient to advanced care. But the procedures that can be performed could be critically important, and you should be ready to quickly react.

CARDIAC ISSUES

Cardiac-related incidents are the leading killer among adults in the United States, followed closely by cancer, and then the mortality rates fall off sharply for the remaining causes of adult death. Statistically, heart attacks are most likely to occur when there are certain relevant risk factors present, such as age (men over 45 and women over 55), family history of cardiac issues, high blood pressure, smoking, and lack of physical activity, among others. The best way to reduce your risk of a heart attack is to reduce your controllable risk factors. There's not much you can do about age, sex, or family history, but by treating high blood pressure, quitting smoking, and leading an active lifestyle, you can greatly reduce your risk.

One of the leading symptoms of a cardiac issue is chest pain. The U.S. *Special Operations Forces Medical Handbook* states that while chest pain is a definite indication of a cardiac issue, it is not an absolute indication of a heart attack, much as other symptoms with the absence of chest pain are not an absolute indication of no heart attack. Pain, "squeezing," or pressure in the chest could be something as benign as stress or heartburn, but should be treated as a cardiac issue until it can be definitively ruled out.

Signs and Symptoms

Note that not all these signs or symptoms need to be present. A cardiac incident could present as any combination of the following:

+ Chest pain, heaviness, squeezing, pressure, or burning in the chest

+ Shortness of breath

+ Pain in the jaw, back, or neck

+ Light-headedness

+ Nausea

+ Vomiting

+ Sweating

Treatment

If you identify a potential cardiac issue:

+ Call 911 if that is an option. If not, follow treatment steps until help arrives.

+ Place the patient in a comfortable position.

+ Loosen any tight or restrictive clothing.

+ If available, have the patient chew two baby aspirin.

+ If the patient has prescribed nitroglycerin tablets, have them place one under their tongue.

+ Monitor ABCs and be prepared to administer CPR if needed.

SEIZURES

Simply put, seizures are an interruption of electrical activity in the brain. They are caused by a variety of factors and can be one of the more frightening medical emergencies to witness. Fortunately, in most cases, seizures cause no damage or long-term effects. Seizure disorders are relatively common and most are treated by medication. Occasionally, someone with a known seizure disorder will experience one, possibly indicating that they, under a doctor's orders, need to adjust their medication.

Tonic-clonic (grand mal) seizures can be one of the scarier seizures to observe and potentially the most dangerous. A tonic-clonic seizure happens in two phases. In the first (tonic) phase, typically lasting less than 60 seconds, the victim falls to the ground, eyes roll back in their head, muscles contract and back arches, and they may make a gurgling sound. The second phase (clonic) happens as the muscles begin to spasm. Extremities and the head will flex and then relax, sometimes violently. The frequency of the spasms will reduce over the next one to two minutes. A tonic-clonic seizure could occur for a variety of reasons, but the field treatment is the same as for other seizures.

A febrile seizure is common, particularly in children under the age of six. The core temperature will spike rapidly, often to above 102°F (39°C), causing the body to convulse. This can be a frightening situation, especially for new parents, but these seizures rarely are harmful or cause long-term issues.

The most common reasons for seizures are:

Epilepsy: This is a neurological condition caused by malfunctioning brain cells.

Head injury: Trauma to the brain can often result in a seizure, and this should be considered a critical medical emergency.

Core temperature: As a person's internal temperature rises, they become at risk, often around 104°F (40°C) or higher, for a febrile seizure.

Stroke: When there is a blockage of blood flow in the brain (a stroke), the patient can experience a seizure.

Signs and Symptoms

+ Convulsions and jerky movements

+ Unconsciousness

+ Stiffness and rigidity

+ Loss of muscle tone

Most people are familiar with what it looks like when someone experiences a seizure. The victim often falls to the ground and begins to shake or convulse violently. Most seizures last less than 60 seconds and some can last as few as 10 seconds. The patient may begin to secrete fluid, including blood, from the mouth. This is the most common seizure, although it is completely possible to have a seizure and experience no loss of consciousness or convulsions. Some seizures will cause the person to simply stare into space and be completely unresponsive for a brief period of time.

Once the seizure is finished, the person will go into a postictal state, or altered state of consciousness. The patient is usually tired, confused, and may have a headache. They may have no memory of the seizure or the events leading up to it. The postictal state can last anywhere from 5 to 15 minutes, or longer on rare occasions. This is the recovery period of the brain.

Treatment

In case of a suspected seizure, do the following:

+ Call 911 if that is an option. If not, follow treatment steps until help arrives.

+ Help the patient to the ground if possible.

+ Clear away things that may injure the person during their convulsions.

+ Place victim on their side to allow fluid to exit the mouth.

+ If possible, put a pad under their head to prevent them from hurting themselves.

+ Make the patient comfortable.

+ After the seizure is over, check the patient for injuries.

DO NOT:

+ Put anything in the patient's mouth. (A common misconception is that they may swallow their tongue. This isn't true.)

+ Attempt to restrain the person.

+ Offer food or drink until they can support their own airway.

DIABETIC EMERGENCIES

Diabetes is a disease that affects how your body uses glucose (blood sugar). Glucose is a main source of fuel for your brain and a significant source of energy for your cells. Being able to properly process blood sugar is extremely important. According to the American Diabetes Association (ADA), there were 29.1 million Americans with diabetes in 2012, and they report 1.4 million Americans are diagnosed every year. The U.S. *Special Operations Forces Medical Handbook* states that diabetes is the most common disease of the endocrine system. It is a common, yet often easily treatable, disease. There are two kinds of diabetes, type 1 and type 2.

Type 1 diabetes: The body breaks down sugars and starches you eat into simple sugar (glucose) that it uses for energy. In type 1 diabetes, the body does not produce insulin, which helps the sugar absorb from the bloodstream to the cells. Most type 1 diabetics have an insulin pump or give themselves daily insulin shots.

Type 2 diabetes: Type 2 diabetics create insulin, but it is not used correctly and the body is unable to regulate glucose levels properly. Type 2 is the most common type of diabetes and is usually controlled with exercise and diet.

Signs and Symptoms

When the glucose level of someone with diabetes gets too high or too low, it can become a medical emergency. The first step in determining how to treat a diabetic emergency is figuring out if their blood sugar is too low (hypoglycemia) or too high (hyperglycemia). Here are a few signs and symptoms to identify:

Hypoglycemia:

+ Weakness

+ Hunger

+ Confusion

+ Irrational behavior

+ Sweating

+ Rapid pulse

+ Insulin in their possession

+ Medical ID bracelet declaring the person as diabetic

Hyperglycemia:

+ Warm, dry skin

+ Rapid breathing

+ Rapid pulse

+ Sweet, fruity breath

+ Extreme thirst

+ Drowsiness

+ Trembling

+ Diminishing level of consciousness

+ Medical ID bracelet declaring the person as diabetic

Treatment

Hypoglycemia:

+ If the patient cannot support their own airway (for example, if they are unconscious) *do not* try to force food or drink into them. Call 911 and monitor their ABCs. Until advanced medical care can be obtained, follow treatment steps.

+ If the patient is conscious, have them lie down.

+ If they carry glucose gel, have them consume it.

+ Have the patient consume something substantial and sugary (fruit juice, peanut butter and jelly, etc.).

+ If they show signs of improvement, have them continue to eat.

+ Help them check their glucose level if they have a testing kit available.

+ If they don't show signs of improvement, monitor their ABCs and provide corrective care as needed.

Hyperglycemia:

+ Call 911 if that is an option. If not, try to get the patient to advanced medical care.

+ Monitor their ABCs.

There is little that can be done for a patient with high blood sugar in the field. They are in need of IV fluid and advanced medical care. If you do not know if they have high or low blood sugar, give them a sugary drink or food. If their blood sugar is low, this should improve their condition. If their blood sugar is high, it is unlikely to make the condition worse.

CHAPTER 12

CHEMICAL, BIOLOGICAL, RADIOLOGICAL, AND NUCLEAR FIRST AID

The *US Army Survival Manual* tells us that nuclear, chemical, and biological weapons have become potential realities on any modern battlefield. Recent conflicts in Afghanistan, Cambodia, and other areas have involved the use of chemical and biological weapons. The warfighting doctrine of the NATO and Warsaw Pact nations addresses the use of both nuclear and chemical weapons. This is not only an issue for foreign soil—it is very much a domestic concern as well. Nuclear, biological, and chemical terrorism is on the rise and is not specific to nations at war. With the ease of access to unlimited information, it isn't difficult for anyone with a little bit of determination to—either by intent or accident—create a deadly problem.

The potential use of these weapons intensifies the problems of survival because of the serious dangers posed by either radioactive fallout or contamination produced by persistent biological or chemical agents. You must use special precautions if you expect to survive these man-made hazards. If you are subjected to any of the effects of nuclear, chemical, or biological warfare, the survival procedures recommended here may save your life. This chapter presents some background information on each type of hazard so that you may better understand its true nature. Awareness of the hazards, knowledge of this chapter, and application of common sense should keep you alive. As you'll read, the best defense is time, distance, and shielding, but when those aren't an option, you should know what to do.

CHEMICAL ENVIRONMENTS

Often, when someone hears the word "chemical," they instantly think of fluid, but a chemical can come in other forms, such as a powder or gas. Chemicals are common, and are created, transported, and used every day. As long as they are safely contained, there isn't an issue. It's only when they breach their container or they are manipulated to cause damage that troubles arise. Chemicals can be immensely problematic in certain industries during a natural disaster, and even as an act of war or terrorism because of their ability to create a large scale hazardous materials spill. A chemical can create extreme trouble in any type of survival situation, but you can overcome the problems with the proper equipment, knowledge, and training.

Chemical agents are grouped according to their effect on the body, based on the primary organ system affected by exposure:

+ Nerve agents (example: sarin, VX)

+ Blood agents (example: hydrogen cyanide)

+ Vesicants or blistering agents (example: mustard gas, lewisite)

+ Lung or choking agents (example: chlorine, phosgene)

SIGNS AND SYMPTOMS

The best method for detecting chemical agents is to use a chemical agent detector. Most people don't have one, but if you do, use it. However, in a survival situation, you'll most likely have to rely solely on the use of all of your physical senses. You must be alert and be able to detect any clues indicating the use of chemical warfare. One of the most dangerous aspects of chemical agents is that they are insidious, often giving no warning that they're causing damage to your body.

Indicators of the presence of chemical agents include:

+ Tears

+ Difficulty breathing

+ Nausea

+ Choking

+ Itching

+ Coughing

+ Dizziness

+ Convulsions

The U.S. Air Force's *Self Aid and Buddy Care Instructor Handbook* explains that NATO defines a chemical agent as "a chemical which is intended for use in military operations to kill, seriously injure, or incapacitate man because of its physiological effects." Unfortunately, chemical agents are often difficult to identify. With agents that are very hard to detect, you must watch for symptoms in fellow survivors. As signs and symptoms begin to appear, you should pay close attention to your environment. Your surroundings will provide valuable clues to the presence of chemical agents, such as dead animals, sick people, or people and animals displaying abnormal behavior. With the absence of a detector that can alert you of a specific chemical's presence, you must rely on your surroundings and your senses.

Your sense of smell may alert you to some chemical agents, but most will be odorless. The odor of newly cut grass or musty hay may indicate the presence of choking agents. A smell of almonds may indicate blood agents. Sight can help you detect chemical agents, as many chemical agents in the solid or liquid state have some color. In the vapor state, you can see some chemical agents as a mist or thin fog immediately after the bomb or shell bursts. By watching for symptoms in others and by observing delivery means, you may be able to have some warning of chemical agents.

Irritation in the nose or eyes, or on the skin, is an urgent warning to protect your body from chemical agents. Additionally, a strange taste in food, water, or cigarettes may serve as a warning that they have been contaminated. Other indicators are:

+ Drooling/runny nose

+ Tightness in the chest

+ Wheezing, coughing, or difficulty breathing

+ Confusion

+ Red, teary eyes

+ Vomiting

+ Convulsions

+ Loss of bladder/bowels control

+ Unconsciousness

PREVENTION

As a survivor, always use the following general steps, in the order listed, to protect yourself from a chemical attack:

1. Use personal protective equipment (PPE).

2. Give quick and correct self-aid when contaminated.

3. Avoid areas where chemical agents exist.

4. Decontaminate your equipment and body as soon as possible.

If you are in close proximity to a chemical leak or attack, your only real chance to avoid injury or death is to have PPE. Without it, you have almost zero protection against the chemical. The detection of chemical agents and avoiding contaminated areas is extremely important to your survival. Avoidance is your best possible defense, but unfortunately, you don't often get that option. Since you're in a survival situation, avoid contaminated areas at all costs. If you do become contaminated, decontaminate yourself as soon as possible using proper procedures. Try to remain uphill and upwind of the chemical. If you find yourself in a contaminated area, try to move out of the area as fast as possible. Travel upwind or crosswind and uphill if possible.

TREATMENT

1. Don appropriate PPE.

2. Safely remove the patient from the hazard.

3. Decontaminate the patient according to what agent they were exposed to.

4. If they are available, and you are trained to use them, you can administer Mark 1, ATNAA (Antidote Treatment, Nerve Agent, Autoinjector), or CANA (Convulsant Antidote for Nerve Agent). These are part of a nerve agent antidote kit, and should be injected into the outer (lateral) thigh muscle of most patients. If the patient is particularly thin, the injection should be done in the upper lateral part of the buttocks. Only use a nerve agent antidote kit if you know what you're doing; these are powerful chemicals and can easily do more harm than good.

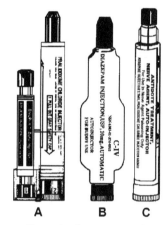

Example of a nerve agent antidote kit: Mark 1 (A), CANA (B), and ATNAA (C).

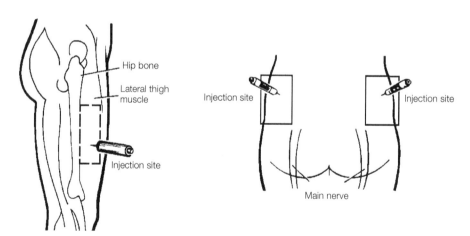

Where to inject nerve agent antidotes

5. Monitor the patient, render corrective care as needed, and evacuate to a medical facility as soon as possible.

BIOLOGICAL AGENTS

Biological agents are microorganisms that can cause disease among personnel, animals, or plants. They can also cause the deterioration of material. These agents fall into two broad categories: pathogens (also called germs) and toxins. Pathogens are living microorganisms such as bacteria, fungi, and viruses that cause lethal or incapacitating diseases. Toxins are poisons that plants, animals, or microorganisms produce naturally. Possible biological warfare toxins include a variety of neurotoxic (affecting the central nervous system) and cytotoxic (causing cell death) compounds.

Germs: Germs are living organisms, the *US Army Survival Manual* tells us. Some nations have figured out how to weaponize them. If inhaled into the lungs, germs can start an infection. Because germs are so small and weigh so little, the wind can spread them over great distances and you can breathe them in without being aware. Buildings and bunkers can trap them, thus causing a higher concentration. Germs do not affect the body immediately. They must multiply inside the body and overcome its defenses, a process called the incubation period. Depending on the germ, incubation periods vary from several hours to several months. Most germs must live within another living organism (host), such as the human body, to survive and grow.

Conditions must be just right for germs to survive. Weather conditions such as wind, rain, cold, and sunlight rapidly kill most germs. Spore-producing agents are a long-term hazard you must neutralize by decontaminating infected areas or personnel. Fortunately, most live agents are not spore-producing. These agents must find a host within roughly a day of their delivery or they die. Germs have three basic routes of entry into your body: through the respiratory tract, through a break in the skin, and through the digestive tract. Symptoms of infection vary according to the disease caused by the germ.

Toxins: Toxins are substances that plants, animals, or germs produce naturally. These toxins, rather than bacteria, are what actually harm people. Botulin, which produces botulism, is an example. Toxins may produce effects similar to those of chemical agents. Toxic victims may not, however, respond to first aid measures used against chemical agents. Toxins enter the body in the same manner as germs. However, some toxins, unlike germs, can penetrate unbroken skin. Symptoms appear almost immediately, since there is no incubation period. Many toxins are extremely lethal, even in very small doses.

SIGNS AND SYMPTOMS

Indicators of the presence of biological agents include:

+ Dizziness

+ Mental confusion

+ Blurred or double vision

+ Numbness or tingling of skin

+ Paralysis

+ Convulsions

+ Rashes or blisters

+ Coughing

+ Fever

+ Aching muscles

+ Tiredness

+ Nausea, vomiting, and/or diarrhea

+ Bleeding from body openings

+ Blood in urine, stool, or saliva

+ Shock

+ Death

PREVENTION

While you must maintain a healthy respect for biological agents, the *US Army Survival Manual* states there is no reason for you to panic. You can reduce your susceptibility to biological agents by doing the following:

+ Maintain current immunizations.

+ Avoid contaminated areas.

+ Control rodents and pests.

+ Use proper first aid measures in the treatment of wounds.

+ Use only safe or properly decontaminated sources of food and water.

+ Ensure that you get enough sleep to prevent a run-down condition.

+ Use proper field sanitation procedures.

+ Practice high standards of personal hygiene.

+ Keep your face covered with some type of cloth.

Dust may contain biological agents; wear some type of mask when dust is in the air. Your clothing and gloves will protect you against bites from most of the insects that carry diseases. Completely button your clothing and tuck your pants tightly into your socks. Wear a chemical protective overgarment, if available, as it provides better protection than normal clothing. Covering your skin will also reduce the chance of the agent entering your body through cuts or scratches.

Personal hygiene is extremely important. Bathe with soap and water whenever possible. Use germicidal soap, if available. Wash your hair and body thoroughly, and clean under your fingernails. Clean your teeth, gums, tongue, and the roof of your mouth frequently. Wash your clothing in hot, soapy water if you can. If you cannot wash your clothing, lay it out in an area of bright sunlight, and allow the light to kill the microorganisms. After a toxin attack, decontaminate yourself using whatever procedure is appropriate for the toxin. Information on the appropriate procedure, if not readily available, can be obtained by doing research on the particular toxin. One resource commonly used by emergency responders is the *Emergency Response Guidebook,* made available to the public by the U.S. Department of Transportation.

TREATMENT

1. Don appropriate PPE.

2. Safely remove patient from hazard.

3. Decontaminate the patient according to what agent they were exposed to.

4. If they are available, and you are trained to use them, you can administer Mark 1 or CANA (part of nerve agent antidote kits).

5. Monitor the patient, render corrective care as needed, and evacuate to a medical facility as soon as possible.

RADIOLOGICAL AGENTS

Radiation is the transmission of energy and is a part of our everyday lives. We even enjoy the light and warmth of radiation in the form of sunshine. Radiation occurs naturally in our environment but can also be artificially created (it's commonly used in X-rays and in the treatment of diseases). However, radiation can be useful or deadly depending on the type of radiation and the precautions in place. When someone receives a dangerous dose of radiation, there are consequences both inside and outside of the body.

External hazards: Highly penetrating gamma radiation or the less penetrating beta radiation that causes burns can cause external damage, producing overall irradiation and beta burns. Treat external radiation burns as you would any other external burn.

Internal hazards: The entry of alpha or beta radiation—emitting particles into the body can cause internal damage. The internal hazard results in irradiation of critical organs such as the gastrointestinal tract, thyroid gland, and bone marrow. A very small amount of radioactive material can cause extreme damage to these and other internal organs. The internal hazard can enter the body either through consumption of contaminated water or food, or by absorption through cuts or abrasions. Material that enters the body through breathing presents only a minor hazard. You can greatly reduce the internal radiation hazard by using good personal hygiene and carefully decontaminating your food and water.

SIGNS AND SYMPTOMS

The effects of radiation on the human body can be broadly classified as either chronic or acute.

Chronic effects: Those that occur some years after exposure to radiation. Examples are cancer and genetic defects. Chronic effects are of minor concern insofar as they don't affect your immediate survival in a radioactive environment.

Acute effects: These are of primary importance to your survival. Some acute effects occur within hours after exposure to radiation. These effects result from the radiation's direct physical damage to tissue. Radiation sickness and beta burns are examples of acute effects. Penetrating beta rays cause radiation burns; the wounds are similar to fire burns.

The extent of physical damage depends mainly on the part of the body exposed to radiation and how long it was exposed, as well as its ability to recover. The brain and kidneys have little recovery capability. Other parts, such as the skin and bone marrow, have a great ability to recover from damage.

Indicators of the presence of radiation include:

+ Nausea

+ Diarrhea

+ Vomiting

+ Fatigue

+ Weakness

+ Hair loss

PREVENTION

Knowledge of the radiation hazards discussed earlier is extremely important to surviving in a fallout area. It's also critical to know how to protect yourself from the most dangerous form of residual radiation: penetrating external radiation. The best means you have to protect yourself from penetrating external radiation are time, distance, and shielding.

Time: Time is important to you, as the survivor, in two ways. First, radiation dosages are cumulative. The longer you're exposed to a radioactive source, the greater the dose you will receive. Obviously, you should spend as little time in a radioactive area as possible. Second, radioactivity decreases or decays over time. This concept is known as radioactive half-life, meaning that a radioactive element decays or loses half of its radioactivity within a certain time. Even an untrained person should realize that the greatest hazard from fallout occurs immediately after detonation, and that the hazard decreases quickly over a relatively short period. As a survivor, try to avoid fallout areas until the radioactivity decays to safe levels. If you can avoid fallout areas long enough for most of the radioactivity to decay, you increase your chance of survival.

Distance: Distance provides very effective protection against penetrating gamma radiation because radiation intensity decreases as a square of the distance from the source. Simply stated, by increasing your distance from a source of radiation, you decrease the radiation dose you receive.

Shielding: This is the most important method of protection from penetrating radiation. Of the three countermeasures against penetrating radiation, it provides the greatest protection and is the easiest to use under survival conditions. Therefore, it is the most desirable method. Shielding actually works by absorbing or weakening the penetrating radiation, thereby reducing the amount of radiation reaching your body. The denser the material, the better the shielding effect.

+ Alpha particles can be shielded by a piece of paper.

+ Beta particles can be shielded by a layer of clothing.

+ Gamma rays can be shielded by lead, iron, or concrete.

If one method of shielding is not possible, use the other two methods to the maximum extent practical.

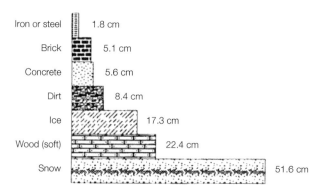

Thickness of materials needed to reduce residual gamma radiation transmission by 50 percent

TREATMENT

The *US Army Survival Manual* states the following:

> *Don't panic if you experience nausea and symptoms of radiation sickness. Your main danger from radiation sickness is infection. There is no first aid for this sickness. Resting, drinking fluids, taking any medicine that prevents vomiting, maintaining your food intake, and preventing additional exposure will help avoid infection and aid recovery. Even small doses of radiation can cause these symptoms, which may disappear in a short time.*

NUCLEAR ENVIRONMENTS

Most injuries in the nuclear environment result from the initial nuclear effects of the detonation. These injuries are classified as blast, thermal, or radiation injuries. Further radiation injuries may occur if you do not take proper precautions against fallout. Individuals in the area near a nuclear explosion will probably suffer a combination of all three types of injuries.

PREVENTION

As with radiation, the best ways to prevent any type of nuclear injury are time, distance, and shielding. Reducing the time a person is exposed reduces the potential risk. Creating as much distance as possible between the source of the nuclear emergency and victims greatly reduces exposure. Lead shielding offers the best protection when a nuclear incident has occurred. The bottom line is to be as far away from a nuclear incident for as long as possible. If someone is exposed, there are several types of injuries associated with a nuclear emergency.

BLAST INJURIES

Blast injuries produced by nuclear weapons are similar to those caused by conventional high-explosive weapons. Blast overpressure can produce collapsed lungs and ruptured internal organs. Projectile wounds occur as the explosion's force hurls debris at you. Large pieces of debris striking you will cause fractured limbs or massive internal injuries. Blast overpressure may throw you long distances, and you will suffer severe injury upon impact with the ground or other objects. Substantial cover and distance from the explosion are the best protection against a blast injury. Cover blast injury wounds as soon as possible to prevent the entry of radioactive dust particles.

Signs and Symptoms

+ Fractures

+ Lacerations

+ Burns

+ Penetrating injuries

+ Head injuries

+ Amputations

+ Asthma or other breathing problems

Treatment

1. Monitor ABCs.

2. Control bleeding.

3. Manage fractures.

THERMAL INJURIES

The heat and light the nuclear fireball emits cause thermal injuries. First, second, or third degree burns may result. Flash blindness can also occur. This blindness may be permanent or temporary depending on the degree of exposure of the eyes. Substantial cover and distance from the explosion can prevent thermal injuries, and clothing will provide significant protection. Cover as much exposed skin as possible before a nuclear explosion. First aid for thermal injuries is the same as first aid for burns. Cover open burns (second or third degree) to prevent the entry of radioactive particles. Wash all burns before covering.

Signs and Symptoms

+ Red skin

+ Pain

+ Blisters

+ Swelling

+ White or charred skin

Treatment

Treat the burn according to the outlined burn procedures starting on page 67.

RADIATION INJURIES

During a nuclear incident, neutrons, gamma radiation, alpha radiation, and beta radiation can cause radiation injuries. Neutrons are high-speed, extremely penetrating particles that actually smash cells within your body. Gamma radiation is similar to X-rays and is also a highly penetrating radiation. During the initial fireball stage of a nuclear detonation, gamma radiation and neutrons are the most serious threats. Beta and alpha radiation are radioactive particles normally associated with radioactive dust from fallout. They are short-range particles, and you can easily protect yourself against them if you take precautions.

Signs and Symptoms

+ Nausea/vomiting

+ Diarrhea

+ Headache

+ Fever

+ Dizziness

+ Fatigue

+ Hair loss

Treatment

1. Remove contaminated clothing.

2. Wash affected skin with soap and water.

3. Monitor ABCs.

4. Evacuate the patient as soon as possible.

GENERAL DECONTAMINATION PROCEDURES

Every hazardous material has a specific decontamination procedure that should be followed if exposure occurs. If you have the Material Safety Data Sheet (MSDS) or the Safety Data Sheet (SDS) that is required to accompany all hazardous materials, follow the specific decontamination procedures outlined on the sheet. One method, called gross decontamination, can be applied in an emergency situation when you don't know the specific chemical present or its correct decontamination procedures.

1. Don PPE—you must wear gloves at a minimum.

2. For nuclear or biological agents, rinse off the victim with a garden hose prior to removing their clothing.

3. Blot chemical agents from the exposed skin immediately, using baby wipes or a wet towel. Brush off any dry products or large chunks with a brush, ideally one with a long handle.

4. Strip off all the patient's clothing.

5. Flush the affected area with large amounts of water, working from the top down.

6. Cover the patient and seek immediate medical intervention as soon as it is available.

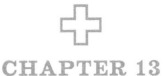

CHAPTER 13
SPECIFIC CLIMATE SURVIVAL

Basic first aid procedures do not vary much regardless of time, place, or conditions. Fracture management and bleeding control procedures are basically the same in every environment. But there are some injuries and illnesses that are more prevalent in some certain climates. You're more likely to treat heatstroke in a hot, arid climate as opposed to a cold, mountainous one.

When placed in these conditions, whether by choice or by a catastrophic event, you are typically a long way from receiving help. There are certain priorities you must have for survival: food, water, shelter, fire, first aid, and distress signals. Depending on the climate you're in, these priorities vary in their importance. For example, in a cold environment, you'll want to build a shelter and fire to warm up and protect yourself from the cold before you make traps and snares to get food or create a means to signal friendly aircraft. If someone is injured, first aid has top priority no matter what climate you're in.

As you may have gathered from previous chapters, a big part of survival medicine is prevention. Many conditions are difficult to treat without a medical professional, and so it's best to try to avoid them completely. In order to do so, you must be able to meet all basic survival priorities. For example, there's no need to treat frostbite if you're able to keep your body warm and protected from the elements. This is why this chapter, though it focuses on survival techniques rather than medical care, is included in this book. Knowing how to survive in different climates will help you avoid and prevent many potential medical conditions.

This chapter will focus on specific procedures based on U.S. military field manuals for survival in a variety of climates. Military survival manuals dedicate hundreds of pages to each specific climate, and years of training are devoted to the subject. The content in this chapter is in no way intended to make you an expert. It will provide a general safety awareness that hopefully will inspire you to do more research specific to each climate and the skills needed to survive there.

SURVIVAL IN ALL ENVIRONMENTS

Some survival knowledge and skills apply to nearly all kinds of environments. When reading about survival information specific to certain biomes, know that these general tips still apply.

FIRE

The ability to make fire is important in any environment. Whether you use it for cooking food, purifying water, signaling for help, or keeping warm, having the means and the ability to make fire is extremely valuable.

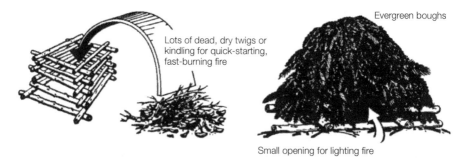

Lots of dead, dry twigs or kindling for quick-starting, fast-burning fire

Evergreen boughs

Small opening for lighting fire

How to use fire to create a signal

The fastest and easiest way to create a fire in any environment is to pack in your own fuel and ignition source. Portable camping stoves or cans of Sterno (jellied alcohol) will ignite easily and burn readily. There are also smaller, more compact sources (such as fuel tablets like hexamine and trioxane) that will burn for several minutes, allowing you ample opportunity to turn a small fire into a larger, more functional one. Finally, candles, hurricane lamps, or road flares can be extremely useful for light, signaling for help, or maintaining a small fire that can be turned into a larger one.

If fuel or oil is available from a wrecked vehicle or downed aircraft, use it. Leave the fuel in the tank for storage, drawing on the supply only as you need it. Oil congeals in extremely cold temperatures; therefore, if you're in a cold environment, drain the fuel from the vehicle or aircraft while it's still warm, and only if there is no danger of explosion or fire.

If you're not fortunate enough to have fuel with you, you'll need to find natural sources in the immediate area. These will vary depending on the environment, but you should be able to locate some kind of natural material that will easily burn. Try to bundle or twist the material into a large, solid mass to create slower burning, more productive fuel. If you have the option, avoid using any plants, dead or alive, that are being used as homes by wildlife. But if it's a survival situation, you must do what you have to.

You will obviously need an ignition source for your fire. A lighter, matches, flint and steel, a magnesium block, or a flare are the easiest ways to create fire. One potential problem with matches is moisture. If they get wet, they become very difficult to ignite. There a few methods that may help you if your matches are wet:

+ Roll a damp match in your hair. Static electricity can help it to dry.

+ Dismantle a flashlight and put the match in the concave reflective piece where the light bulb typically goes. Aim it toward the sun. If you do this long enough, the match may ignite.

+ Strike the match at a sharp angle rather than at the typical perpendicular angle.

+ Have another long-burning object or tinder ready to light because the match may not remain lit for long.

If you don't have any fire starters available to you, you aren't out of options. There are many ways to start a fire, but building one without matches or a lighter takes skill and practice. You can use a lens to magnify the sun's rays, metal to reflect and focus sun rays, friction from sticks (fire-plow method), and a variety of other methods. The time to learn this is *not* when the need arises. Research several ways to start a fire now, and practice at home when your life doesn't depend on it.

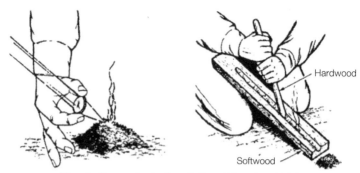

Fire-starting methods: lens (left) and fire-plow (right)

If you've practiced your fire-starting skills and you are able to create fire, you won't want to lose it. The military suggests ways to "carry" a fire. By carrying a fire, you can safely bring a smoldering material with you, making the next fire you build far simpler. To carry a fire:

1. Locate a non-combustible receptacle (aluminum can, tin can, metal bucket, etc.).

2. Poke holes in the sides to allow airflow.

3. Place a slow-burning material such as moss in the bottom.

4. Place embers on top of the moss.

5. Add another layer of slow-burning material on top of the embers.

6. Be careful not to pack the receptacle too tightly or too loosely; this may take some trial and error.

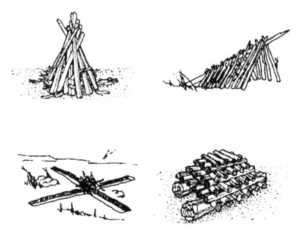

Methods for laying fires: tepee (top left), lean-to (top right),
cross-ditch (bottom left), pyramid (bottom right)

There are many different kinds of fires you can build. One that is particularly useful for cooking food without burning it is the tripod fire. To build one, follow these steps:

1. Locate three sturdy sticks roughly the same length.

2. Lash the sticks together at the top.

3. Tie a fourth, forked stick to the lashing, pointing upward.

4. Suspend a cooking pot by its handle in the upward-pointing fork.

5. Relocate the pot up or down as needed and as the "fork" allows.

WATER

More than three-quarters of your body is composed of fluids. Your body loses fluid as a result of heat, cold, stress, and exertion. To function effectively, you must replace the fluid your body loses. According to the U.S. Army, if the ambient temperature is below 100°F (38°C), you should consume a pint of water every hour; above 100°F (38°C) you should consume a quart every hour. So, one of your first goals in a survival situation is to obtain an adequate supply of water. It's always best to have safe drinking water with you, but if you need to find a source of water, you'll need to be able to identify potable water and know where to find it.

Even if you're able to locate it, however, standing water may not be safe. Pollution, chemicals, and microorganisms, among other things, can contaminate water, making it unsafe for consumption. Extreme thirst will cause you to want to gamble and drink questionable water. This is extremely dangerous and could potentially make a bad situation worse.

A simple water filter can be made with a water bottle, knife, cotton balls or coffee filter, sand, gravel, larger rocks, and a cup. This does not purify dirty water, but it does make it easier to drink. Just follow these simple steps:

1. Cut the bottom off a water bottle.

2. Use a knife to make a small hole in the bottle's cap.

3. Put your cotton or coffee filter through the open bottom of the bottle and push it up to the narrow, capped side of the bottle. Keep the bottle inverted.

4. Add about 2 inches of sand.

5. Add about 2 inches of gravel.

6. Add about 2 inches of larger rocks.

7. Pour water through the large opening using a cup. As it flows from the larger rocks down through the sand, it will be filtered. It will run out of the small hole in the bottle cap, where you can collect it with the cup.

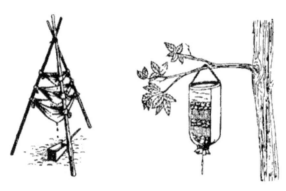

Water filtering systems

If you're unable to locate clean, drinkable water, then you'll need to have the means to purify it. Unless it is a life-or-death situation, all water should be treated before drinking. Better to be safe than sorry. There are many inexpensive water purifiers on the market today that can be easily packed into your bag, such as iodine or chlorine tablets, or UV sticks. However, if you find yourself without the benefit of a commercial water purifier, you'll need the skills to make contaminated water drinkable. Boiling water is the easiest and one of the most effective ways to decontaminate water in the wilderness. Bringing the water to a boil (212°F/100°C) should kill all pathogens. Military survival manuals recommend boiling the water for at least one minute, and up to 10 minutes, before cooling and consuming. Boiling can also eliminate some of the distinctive taste left by chlorine or iodine tablets.

Water should also be purified prior to use for wound care due to the high likelihood that it contains bacteria.

There are also a variety of stills you can build in order to collect water. One of the most common and simplest is a solar still. Contrary to popular belief, however, it will not provide enough water to meet the daily requirement.

Solar stills are designed to supplement water reserves. Several stills must be made in order to procure the daily amount of needed water. The *US Marine Corps Summer Survival Course Handbook* gives instructions on how to build both aboveground and belowground solar stills.

Aboveground Solar Still

This device allows the survivor to make water from vegetation. To make the aboveground solar still, locate a sunny slope on which to place the still, a clear plastic bag, green leafy vegetation, and a small rock. Using a 1-gallon zip-top bag instead of a trash bag is a more efficient means of construction.

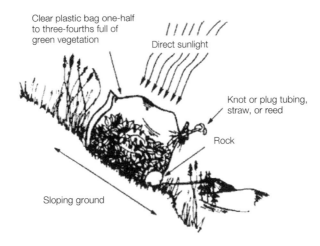

Clear plastic bag one-half to three-fourths full of green vegetation

Direct sunlight

Knot or plug tubing, straw, or reed

Rock

Sloping ground

1. Fill the bag with air by turning the opening into the breeze or by "scooping" air into the bag.

2. Fill the bag one-half to three-fourths full of green leafy vegetation. Be sure to remove all hard sticks or sharp spines that might puncture the bag.

3. Place a small rock or similar item in the bag.

4. Close the bag and tie the mouth securely as close to the end of the bag as possible to keep the maximum amount of air space. If you have a small piece of tubing, small straw, or hollow reed, insert one end in the mouth of the bag before tying it securely. Tie off or plug the tubing so that air will not escape. This tubing will allow you to drain out condensed water without untying the bag.

5. Place the bag, mouth downhill, on a slope in full sunlight. Position the mouth of the bag slightly higher than the low point in the bag so that the rock works itself into the low point.

6. To get the condensed water from the still, loosen the tie and tip the bag so that the collected water drains out. Retie the mouth and reposition the still to allow further condensation.

7. Change the vegetation in the bag after extracting most of the water from it.

Caution: Do not use poisonous vegetation. It will make poisonous liquid.

Belowground Solar Still

Materials for this kind of still consist of a digging stick, clear plastic sheet, container, rock, and drinking tube.

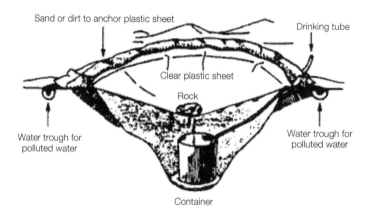

1. Select a site where you believe the soil will contain moisture (such as a dry streambed or a low spot where rainwater has collected). The soil should be easy to dig and should be exposed to sunlight.

2. Dig a bowl-shaped hole about 3 feet across and 2 feet deep.

3. Dig a sump in the center of the hole. The sump depth and perimeter will depend on the size of the container you have to place in it. The bottom of the sump should allow the container to stand upright.

4. Anchor the tubing to the container's bottom by forming a loose overhand knot in the tubing. Extend the unanchored end of the tubing up, over, and beyond the lip of the hole.

5. Place the plastic sheet over the hole, covering its edges with soil to hold it in place. Place a rock in the center of the plastic sheet.

6. Lower the plastic sheet into the hole until it is about 18 inches below ground level. Make sure the cone's apex is directly over the container. Ensure the plastic does not touch the sides of the hole, because the earth will absorb the moisture.

7. Add more soil on the edges of the plastic to hold it securely and prevent moisture loss.

8. Plug the tube when not in use so that moisture will not evaporate.

9. Plants can be placed in the hole as a moisture source. If so, dig out additional soil from the sides.

10. If polluted water is the only moisture source, dig a small trough, about 10 inches deep and 3 inches wide, outside the hole about 10 inches from the still's lip. Pour the polluted water in the trough. Ensure you do not spill any polluted water around the rim of the hole where the plastic touches the soil. The trough holds the polluted water and the soil filters it as the still draws it. This process works well when the only water source is salt water.

Note: Three stills may be needed to meet the individual daily water intake you will require. These can be a combination of different types of stills.

SHELTER

Any type of shelter, whether it is a permanent building, tentage, or an expedient shelter, must meet six basic criteria to be safe and effective:

+ Drying facility

+ Free from natural hazards

+ Heat retention

+ Protection from the elements

+ Stable

+ Ventilation

When all six criteria are met, you likely have a functional and safe shelter. It must provide protection from rain, snow, wind, and sun. It must have insulation properties to keep the warmth in and cold out. It must allow for ventilation to prevent the accumulation of carbon monoxide and carbon dioxide. It must have an area to dry wet clothing. It should not be built in areas that have the potential for a flood, fire, avalanche, or any other disaster, and it should be stable enough to withstand dangerous weather conditions.

These are common mistakes you should avoid.

DO NOT:

+ Assume you don't need shelter—you do

+ Build in a flood or avalanche zone

+ Build on a game trail

+ Build near a lone tree—it could attract lightning

+ Build under a dead tree

+ Build in an especially low or high spot—use natural protection

+ Light a fire in your shelter unless you are certain there is adequate ventilation

Natural Shelters

Natural shelters are usually the preferred type because they take less time and materials to construct. You can often find a cave or rock overhang to provide protection. You should build a wall of rocks, logs, or branches across the open sides for additional shelter. Another option is to locate a hollow log that can be cleaned or dug out. You can then lay a poncho or tarp across the opening to offer protection. Look for a natural shelter that meets the six basic criteria (see page 137) and is preferably close to a water source.

Natural shelters do have a few inherent hazards. First of all, if it is a suitable shelter, you're likely not the only creature to think so. Animals may already inhabit the shelter. The animal itself is one of several concerns, which also include disease from animal waste and decaying carcasses. Natural shelters also typically lack adequate ventilation, making it dangerous to build a fire for heating or cooking. In fact, it could be a deadly mistake to build a fire in a shelter without adequate ventilation. There are other considerations with natural shelters such as natural gas pockets and just general instability. In order to conserve heat, your ideal shelter will be only big enough for you, your things, and what you need to do. Choose your natural shelter carefully.

Man-made Shelters

There are many configurations of man-made shelters that can be used. The *US Army Survival Manual* states that your environment and the equipment you carry with you will determine the type of shelter you can build. Unused man-made structures found in urban or rural environments, such as houses, sheds, or barns, may also provide shelter.

To maximize a shelter's effectiveness, you should take into consideration the following prior to construction:

+ Group size

+ Reduced living area (heat conservation)

+ Avoid exposed hilltops, valley floors, moist ground, and avalanche paths

+ Create a thermal shelter by applying snow to the roof and sides of the shelter

+ Close proximity to water, firewood, and a signaling location

+ Time and effort needed to construct the shelter

+ Does it provide adequate protection from the elements?

+ Do you have the means to build the shelter?

+ Do you have the types and amount of materials needed to build the shelter?

Assuming you have the appropriate materials and landmarks, any type of shelter can be constructed just about anywhere. The following shelter, however, is so basic and versatile that its uses are limited only by your imagination and the materials available. See any particular climate in this chapter for climate-specific shelters.

Poncho shelter: This is one of the easiest shelters to construct. Materials needed for construction are cord and any water-repellent material (i.e., poncho, parachute, tarp). It should be one of the first types of shelter considered if planning a short stay in any one place.

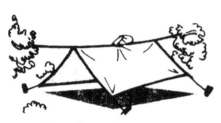

Hasty Shelter-Canopy Fashion

A hasty shelter is made by suspending a poncho from low underbush. Due to its simplicity, it can be easily erected at night, especially if heavy strings have already been tied to the corners of the poncho.

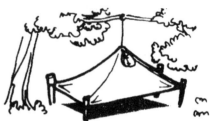

Hasty Shelter-Canopy Fashion

This is another hasty shelter pitched canopy fashion.

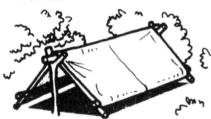

Poncho and Spreader Bars

This is a hasty shelter using a poncho and two branches for spreader bars.

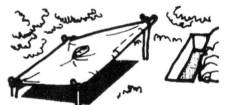

Low Silhouette Shelter

This low silhouette shelter can be used while improving fighting positions. It can be lowered by removing the front upright supports.

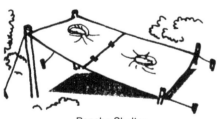

Poncho Shelter

Two ponchos fastened together will shelter four adults from the rain. Extra ponchos can be used as ground sheets.

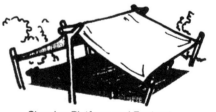

Sleeping Platform and Footrest

This type of shelter may be used for a longer stay in more secure areas. A sleeping platform and footrest protect from dampness and insects.

1. Find the center of the water-repellent material by folding it in half along its long axis.

2. Suspend the center points of the two ends using cordage.

3. Stake the four corners down with sticks or rocks.

FOOD

You can function for a time without food, but that doesn't mean you should. Your strength, spirit, and ability to think rationally will decrease the longer you go without food. It is best to identify early what type of food is available. Survival experts have devised the Universal Edibility Test in order to determine if a plant is edible or toxic. There are over 700 varieties of poisonous plants in the United States and Canada alone. Most of the time that fact is merely interesting, but in a survival scenario it becomes a serious concern. The Universal Edibility Test is time-consuming, but in the absence of concrete knowledge, it is the safest way to consume unknown plants.

Universal Edibility Test

1. Separate the plant into its various parts: roots, stems, leaves, buds, and flowers.

2. Test one part of the plant at a time.

3. Smell for strong or acidic odors—a bad smell is a bad sign.

4. Test for contact poisoning—hold the part of the plant against your wrist or inner elbow for several minutes, and wait 15 minutes to see if there's a reaction.

5. If the part has passed the steps above, prepare it the way you plan to eat it—boiling is always a safe option.

6. Touch part of the plant to your lips. Wait 15 minutes to see if there is any itching or burning.

7. If there is no reaction, put a small part of the plant in your mouth and hold it there for 15 minutes. If it tastes bitter or soapy, spit it out.

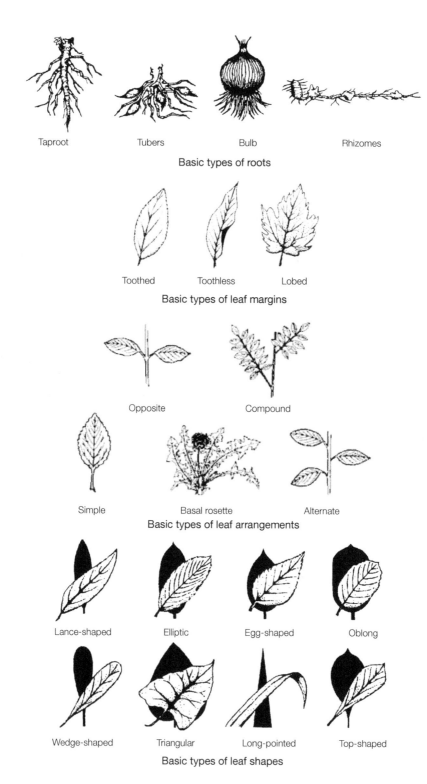

Taproot Tubers Bulb Rhizomes

Basic types of roots

Toothed Toothless Lobed

Basic types of leaf margins

Opposite Compound

Simple Basal rosette Alternate

Basic types of leaf arrangements

Lance-shaped Elliptic Egg-shaped Oblong

Wedge-shaped Triangular Long-pointed Top-shaped

Basic types of leaf shapes

8. If there is no reaction, swallow the bite and wait several hours to see if there is an adverse reaction.

9. If there are no ill effects, it can be assumed that part of the plant is safe to eat. Prepare a small amount (¼ cup) and consume, waiting again for several hours after to feel any adverse effects.

Once you have gathered plants or animals to eat, you'll need to be able to cook them. Any fire will create enough heat to kill bacteria, warm the meat, or boil the water. If you are fortunate enough to have a pot to cook in, you're ahead of most and should certainly use it and keep it clean and secure. If not, you'll have to improvise using whatever you have available.

It is a good idea to have a detailed field guide, particularly for edible plants, such as *The Forager's Harvest: A Guide to Identifying, Harvesting, and Preparing Edible Wild Plants* or the *SAS Survival Handbook,* which can help to safely identify edible plants and avoid dangerous ones.

MEDICINAL PLANTS

In each climate, there are medicinal plants that can be utilized when needed. While many plants and herbs are effective and even used in modern medications to treat a variety of ailments, the *US Army Survival Manual* cautions to "use herbal medicines with extreme care and only when you lack or have limited medical supplies. Some herbal medicines are dangerous and may cause further damage or even death." It's best to do your research and consult a medical professional to check for possible interactions with other medications or allergies.

Further information on survival can be found in the following publications:

+ *SAS Survival Handbook: The Ultimate Guide to Surviving Anywhere* by John "Lofty" Wiseman

+ *The Ultimate Guide to U.S. Army Survival Skills, Tactics, and Techniques* edited by Jay McCullough

+ *Tom Brown's Guide to Wild Edible and Medicinal Plants* by Tom Brown

+ *Camping & Wilderness Survival* by Paul Tawrell

+ *The Prepper's Workbook* by Scott B. Williams and Scott Finazzo

DESERT

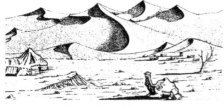

Dune desert terrain

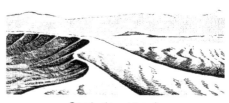

Sandy desert terrain

The word "desert" usually evokes images of an endless panoramic view of fiercely hot, dry sand dunes. But a desert is defined by the amount of moisture a region receives. A desert can be mountainous, flat, jagged, or have rolling sand dunes. For example, Antarctica is actually a desert, receiving less than 10 inches of precipitation per year. However, for the purposes of this section, we'll stick to the typical image of a desert: a barren wasteland that is hostile to any living thing with almost no vegetation that could support human life. Deserts cover one-fifth of the earth's land masses.

Surviving in an arid area depends on what you know and how prepared you are for the environmental conditions you will face. Those who find themselves in harsh desert conditions are seriously challenged. Certain measures must be taken to ensure survival. If you live in or plan to be in a desert environment, determine what equipment you'll need, the tactics you'll use, and the environment's impact on them and you. The *US Army Survival Manual* characterizes deserts by seven environmental factors that you must consider:

+ Low rainfall

+ Intense sunlight and heat

+ Wide temperature range

+ Sparse vegetation

+ High mineral content near ground surface

+ Sandstorms

+ Mirages

Each of the seven environmental factors can create significant survival and first aid dangers. First aid can be managed by taking survival measures:

being able to make fire, procuring water, finding or building shelter, obtaining food, and being aware of climate-specific hazards.

DESERT HAZARDS

Deserts are notorious for high heat during the day, cold nighttime temperatures, sandstorms, and animal hazards. A desert is a beautiful but unforgiving climate. The potential for injuries is everywhere, from sunburn to dehydration to snakebites or scorpion stings to simple fall hazards in the soft sand and jagged rocks. Being aware of the dangers affords you the ability to try to avoid them.

+ **Sunburn**: Avoid the sun if at all possible during the heat of the day.

+ **Dehydration**: Consume enough water to keep you alive and functioning.

+ **Heat-related injuries**: Limit your exposure to direct sunlight and avoid exerting yourself (see Chapter 7).

+ **Blisters**: Proper footwear is extremely important.

+ **Falls**: Ensure proper footing, especially over difficult terrain.

+ **Spiny vegetation**: Even the smallest spines can be extremely painful.

+ **Bites and stings**: Immediately treat them (see Chapter 10), and watch for anaphylaxis.

+ **Sandstorms**: Eye, skin, and respiratory injuries are significant threats. Sandstorms can occur with little warning and render you paralyzed with the inability to see and difficulty breathing. The driving sand tears at your skin and clothing, leaving you the unwilling recipient of an all-out assault on your body unless you are able to find shelter. The best way to avoid sandstorm injuries is to take the following precautions:

  • Wait it out in a shelter or windbreak.

  • If caught in the open, lay on your side at the base of a dune, hill, or object opposite the wind.

  • Cover all exposed skin.

  • Cover your mouth, nose, and eyes.

- Put on eye protection (goggles—not prescription glasses) if you have it.

- If natural shelter is unavailable, use stones to mark your direction of travel. The storm may change the landscape and disorient you as to which way you were going.

The best way to avoid the worst the desert has to offer comes down to three steps: hydrate, keep out of the sun, and keep cool. The *US Army Survival Manual* states that someone working hard in the sun will require 19 liters (5 gallons) of water a day to maintain normal function. You'll be losing a lot of water in the form of sweat and therefore will need to replenish yourself. Consuming a healthy amount of water will also help maintain a safe core temperature, thus avoiding heat-related illnesses. Finally, stay out of the sun as much as possible. In a survival situation that is easier said than done, but finding shelter wherever you can could mean the difference between life and death.

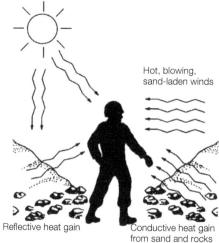

Hot, blowing, sand-laden winds

Reflective heat gain

Conductive heat gain from sand and rocks

Types of heat gain

FIRE IN THE DESERT

Fire is important even in a blistering hot, dry climate such as the desert. You may not necessarily need it, but having the means and the ability to make fire is extremely valuable.

Some natural desert fuel options are:

+ Dry scrub brush

+ Dead cacti

+ Dry grasses (twist them into bunches)

+ Dry donkey, cow, or camel dung

+ Bark from the base of old ocotillos

+ Cottonwood, willow, or acacia branches

+ Abandoned bird or mouse nests

Be aware that creating a fire in a desert environment can be very dangerous. Dry ground cover ignites easily and can quickly spread beyond your ability to extinguish it. Dead cacti and brush also provide homes and shelter for wildlife. You can easily do a lot of damage by not being careful about your fire.

WATER IN THE DESERT

Nothing is more critical to desert survival than water. During World War II, the U.S. Army took steps to prepare soldiers to fight in the extreme heat of North Africa. To condition the soldiers, they instituted "water discipline," which meant that water would become progressively less available during training. Rather than conditioning the soldiers to work in high heat conditions with minimal water, this exercise created hundreds of heat casualties. Desert survival depends on the relationship between ambient temperature, physical activity, and water consumption.

Your body gets rid of excess heat (cools off) by sweating. The warmer your body becomes, whether through work, exercise, or air temperature, the more you sweat. The more you sweat, the more moisture you lose. Sweating is the principal cause of water loss. Drinking water at regular intervals helps your body remain cool and decreases sweating. Even when your water supply is low, sipping water constantly will keep your body cooler and reduce water loss. Conserve your fluids by reducing activity during the heat of day. Use caution if you try to ration your water! By rationing water, you stand a good chance of becoming a heat casualty.

There are a number of ways to locate water in the desert:

+ Cut into vegetation (such as cactus).

  • Locate a barrel cactus (short, spiny, cylindrical with pink or yellow flowers).

- Carefully cut off the top.

- Mash the insides until they are reduced to a pulp.

- Strain the pulp through a thin cloth such as a bandanna or shirt. (If straining the pulp is not an option, suck on it to pull the moisture from it, but do not eat it.)

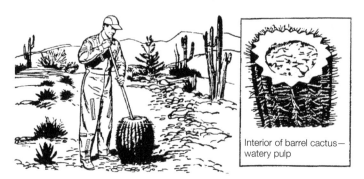

Interior of barrel cactus—watery pulp

+ Dig into moist soil—this may indicate water below the surface.

+ Locate depressions in porous rock.

+ Sop up dew with a dry cloth and suck on it or wring it out into your mouth.

+ Look for seepage in canyon walls.

+ Follow a dry riverbed to its source—water may still exist there. Caution: Following riverbeds may lead you to water, but be careful—rain can fill them with flash floods.

+ Locate cottonwoods or willows, whose water needs are greater than cacti and whose existence may indicate water.

DESERT SHELTERS

A shelter in the desert can be very rudimentary. You basically need something to shade you from the searing daytime sun and to hold in warmth during cold desert nights. The temperature in the shade can be 20 to 40°F cooler than in direct sunlight. Shelter will promote cooling of the body, slow dehydration, and, at night, help reduce the chances for hypothermia.

If you don't have building materials, you must use what is available to you in the desert: sand, rocks, and possibly dry brush. When locating or building a desert shelter, keep these tips in mind:

+ It must provide shade.

+ It will reduce the sun's impact if your shelter has a northern exposure in the Northern Hemisphere and a southern exposure in the Southern Hemisphere.

+ If possible, build your shelter in close proximity to a water source.

+ Do not build your shelter in low spots where a rainstorm will create flash flooding.

+ Avoid using a cool, damp place as a shelter—such spots are favorites of snakes and scorpions.

+ Check your space and continually evaluate for pests and wildlife.

+ The *US Army Survival Manual* states, "In an arid environment, consider the time, effort, and material needed to make a shelter. If you have material such as a poncho, canvas, or parachute, use it along with such terrain features as rock outcroppings, mounds of sand, or a depression between dunes or rocks to make your shelter."

Sandy Area Shelter

1. Build a mound of sand or use the side of a sand dune for one side of the shelter.

2. Anchor one end of the material on top of the mound using sand or other weights.

3. Extend and anchor the other end of the material so it provides the best possible shade.

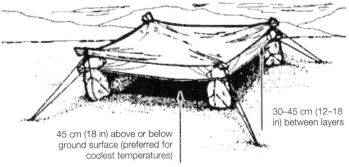

30–45 cm (12–18 in) between layers

45 cm (18 in) above or below ground surface (preferred for coolest temperatures)

Note: If you have enough material, fold it in half and form a 30- to 45-centimeter (about 12- to 18-inch) airspace between the two halves. This airspace will reduce the temperature in the shelter.

Belowground Shelter

A belowground shelter can reduce the midday heat by as much as 30 to 40°F. Building it, however, requires more time and effort than is needed for other shelters. Since your physical effort will make you sweat more and increase dehydration, construct it before the heat of the day.

To make this shelter:

1. Find a low spot or depression between dunes or rocks. If necessary, dig a trench 45 to 60 centimeters (18 to 24 inches) deep and long, and wide enough for you to lie down in comfortably.

2. Pile the sand you take from the trench to form a mound around three sides.

3. On the open end of the trench, dig out more sand so you can get in and out of your shelter easily.

4. Cover the trench with your material.

5. Secure the material in place using sand, rocks, or other weights.

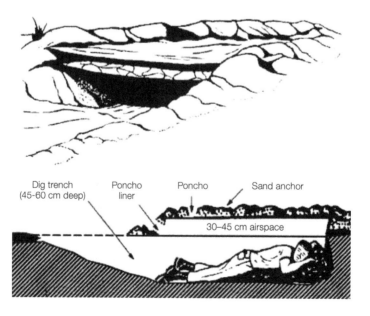

If you have extra material, you can further decrease the midday temperature in the trench by securing the additional material 30 to 45 centimeters (12 to 18 inches) above the first. This layering of the material will reduce the inside temperature. White is the best color to reflect heat; the innermost layer should be of darker material.

If nothing else is available, even sand can be used as a desert shelter. As an insulator, it can keep you either cool or warm. Dig down into the sand and cover your body with it, obviously leaving your face exposed to breathe. Cover your face with a cloth or something to protect it from the sun.

DESERT FOOD

You should expect food to be sparse in the desert. The harsher the desert, the lower the chance for plant or animal life. In some ways, the limited amount of food available in the desert environment can be beneficial. Eating without adequate water speeds up dehydration. Heat also reduces your appetite, so you may not feel as hungry in the desert as you would in other climates. Eating is a secondary need in the desert, far behind water. But you will need to eat to sustain good health and energy.

Desert edibles will depend on the type of desert you're in and they are divided into two categories: plants and animals. Use caution and make sure you can positively identify edible plants. Consuming the wrong plant can cause vomiting (speeding up the dehydration process) or death. Even some edible plants can be difficult to eat unless properly cooked.

Edible Plants in the Desert

+ **Acacia**: Young leaves, flowers, and pods can be eaten raw or cooked.

+ **Agave**: Flowers and flower buds are edible, but boil before eating.

+ **Cactus**: There are dozens of edible varieties. Look for the mature fruit of the prickly pear, organ pipe, saguaro, and cholla cactus.

+ **Date palm**: The fruit is edible if fresh, but very bitter if eaten before it is ripe.

+ **Desert amaranth**: All parts of this plant are edible, but ensure you have removed the sharp spines before eating.

+ **Yucca**: Eat the flowers raw or cooked.

Edible Animals in the Desert

+ **Lizards**: Kill them with a stick or a noose, then skin, gut, and cook.

+ **Snakes**: Stun them with a rock or large stick before killing them. After killing a snake, 1) grip the dead snake firmly behind the head, 2) cut off at least 15 cm (6 in) behind the head, 3) slit belly and remove innards, and 4) skin. Now cook.

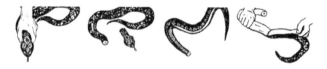

1.   2.

3.   4.

+ **Rabbits**: Like snakes, stun them with a rock or large stick before killing them, then skin, gut, and cook.

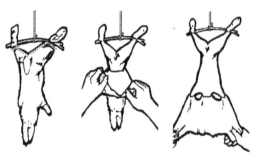

How to skin a rabbit

+ **Insects**: Adults and larvae can be high in protein; for preparation, roast, remove head, legs, and wings, and then eat the body.

+ **Crustaceans**: Located in shallow water along desert shorelines. Some varieties can be eaten raw, but to be safe boil or cook them over a fire. Avoid mollusks from April to October (see the "R rule" on page 166).

DESERT MEDICINAL PLANTS

Desert plants have been used for medicinal purposes for as long as humans have been living in deserts. Some plant remedies are based in lore and have no scientific evidence or proven medical results. Others, though, have been successfully utilized to treat a variety of maladies.

Gumweed: A member of the sunflower family, gumweed stimulates mucous membranes in the treatment of asthma and chronic bronchitis. The floral heads are eaten whole.

Identification:

+ 1 to 3 feet tall with fibrous roots

+ Sawtooth leaves 1 to 3 inches long

+ Yellow flowers 1 inch in diameter

+ Curved bracts around the flower secret a sticky resin

Desert sage: Sage leaves can be chewed to relieve indigestion and gastrointestinal issues, as well as to remedy a sore throat. It's also said the leaves can be brewed into a tea and consumed to help with aches, pains, and gum and mouth diseases.

Identification:

+ 2 to 3 feet tall

+ Two lipped flowers arrange themselves in balls on the stem

+ Purple flowers

+ Flowers bloom from May to July

Yucca: Yucca has been used to reduce high blood pressure and cholesterol. It can also be used as soap and shampoo. The fruits can be boiled or baked, the blossoms can be eaten, and the leaves can be chewed.

Identification:

+ Grayish brown trunk 6 to 12 inches in diameter

+ Grows up to 16 feet tall

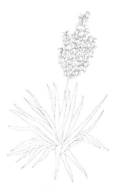

Yucca

+ Bayonet-like leaves

+ Purplish-white, bell-shaped flowers

Agave: Agave has been used as a laxative, an anti-inflammatory, and a diuretic. The leaves can be eaten to treat constipation and gas, and can be a diuretic to assist with urination. The roots can be boiled into a tea to help with pain relief and arthritis.

Identification:

+ Clusters of yellow flowers growing 3 inches across

+ Large rosettes of sharp-toothed leaves

+ Short stem with leaves apparently growing from the root

Prickly pear: The pulp of the prickly pear can be used to calm an uneasy digestive tract. It is believed that the prickly pear also possesses blood sugar–balancing properties that can be helpful for diabetes. The pads can also be cut open and placed on burns or wounds to reduce inflammation.

Identification:

+ Green, flat, pad-like stems

+ Most have yellow, red, or purple flowers

+ Round, furry dots that contain spines

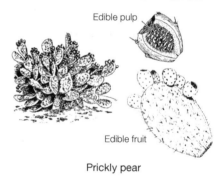

Edible pulp

Edible fruit

Prickly pear

COLD REGIONS

For military purposes, cold regions are defined as those where cold temperatures, unique terrain, and snowfall significantly affect military operations for one month or more each year. About one-quarter of the earth's land mass may be termed "severely cold." Another quarter of the earth is termed "moderately cold." As with the desert, your needs for survival do not change, but the major obstacle that you must overcome does: cold. In addition to temperature, though, you must also factor in the windchill, which is the heat lost from exposed skin due to wind and cold—basically, how cold it actually feels.

It's more difficult to satisfy your basic water, food, and shelter needs in a cold environment than in a warm environment. Even if you have the basic requirements, you must also have adequate protective clothing and the will to survive, which is as important as the basic needs. There have been incidents when trained and well-equipped individuals have not survived cold-weather situations because they lacked the will to live. Conversely, this will has sustained individuals less well-trained and equipped. The military technical bulletin *Prevention and Management of Cold-Weather Injuries* warns that "excessive cold stress degrades physical performance capabilities, significantly impacts morale, and eventually causes cold casualties."

Within the cold-weather regions, you may face two types of environments: wet or dry. Knowing which environment you will face will help you better prepare and survive.

Wet cold-weather environments: Wet cold-weather conditions exist when the average temperature in a 24-hour period is 14°F (–10°C) or above. Characteristics of this condition are freezing during the colder night hours and thawing during the day. Even though the temperatures are warmer in this environment than a dry cold region, the terrain is usually very sloppy due to slush and mud. You must concentrate on protecting yourself from the wet ground and from freezing rain or wet snow.

Dry cold-weather environments: Dry cold-weather conditions exist when the average temperature in a 24-hour period remains below 14°F (–10°C). Even though the temperatures in this environment are much lower than normal, you do not have to contend with the freezing and thawing. In these conditions, you need more layers of inner clothing to protect you from temperatures as low as –76°F (–60°C). Extremely hazardous conditions exist when wind and low temperature combine.

The key to survival in arctic regions is simply keeping warm and dry. Here are a few tips to help:

+ Wear waterproof clothing.

+ Wear waterproof footwear.

+ Brush off snow before entering your shelter where it will melt and get things wet.

+ Remove layers when you can to prevent sweating.

+ Use a water-repellent and cold-weather sleeping bag with a pad underneath.

+ Use drying racks inside your shelter for clothing.

+ *Never* assume frozen water is safe to traverse.

There are many different items of cold-weather equipment and clothing issued by the U.S. Army and available to the public today. There have been major strides in cold-weather gear over the past decade. Remember, however, that older gear will keep you warm as long as you apply a few cold-weather principles. If the newer types of clothing are available, use them. If not, then your clothing should be entirely wool, with the possible exception of a windbreaker. Not only must you have enough clothing to protect you from the cold, but you must also know how to maximize the warmth you get from it. For example, always keep your head covered. You can lose 40 to 45 percent of body heat from an unprotected head and even more from an unprotected neck, wrists, and ankles. These areas of the body are good radiators of heat and have very little insulating fat. The brain is very susceptible to cold and can stand the least amount of cooling. Because there is much blood circulation in the head, most of which is on the surface, you can lose heat quickly if you do not cover your head.

Estimated wind speed (in MPH)	Actual Thermometer Reading (°F)											
	50	40	30	20	10	0	-10	-20	-30	-40	-50	-60
	Equivalent Chill Temperature (°F)											
Calm	50	40	30	20	10	0	-10	-20	-30	-40	-50	-60
5	48	37	27	16	6	-5	-15	-26	-36	-47	-57	-68
10	40	28	16	4	-9	-24	-33	-46	-58	-70	-83	-95
15	36	22	9	-5	-18	-32	-45	-58	-72	-85	-99	-112
20	32	18	4	-10	-25	-39	-53	-67	-82	-96	-110	-124
25	30	16	0	-15	-29	-44	-59	-74	-88	-104	-118	-133
30	28	13	-2	-18	-33	-48	-63	-79	-94	-109	-125	-140
35	27	11	-4	-21	-35	-51	-67	-82	-98	-113	-129	-145
40	26	10	-6	-21	-37	-53	-69	-85	-100	-116	-132	-148
Wind speeds greater than 40 MPH have little additional effect.	LITTLE DANGER Under 5 hours with dry skin. Maximum danger of false sense of security.				INCREASING DANGER Flesh may freeze within one minute.			GREAT DANGER Flesh may freeze within 30 seconds.				
	Danger from freezing of exposed flesh.											
	Immersion foot (trench foot) may occur at any point on this chart.											

COLD ENVIRONMENT HAZARDS

The colder parts of the planet are full of peril. Temperature is only one of the many dangers that abound in the Arctic. You also have to concern yourself with predators, dehydration, and snowstorms. There are hidden crevices and thin ice that are capable of swallowing you in an instant. Then there's the ever-present risk of frostbite and hypothermia that lurks constantly around you. There are many hazards specific to snow and icy regions that you should be aware of and avoid if possible:

+ **Dehydration**: Even in cold regions, adequate levels of water must be consumed.

+ **Cold-related injuries**: Measures must be taken to ensure all parts of your body maintain a safe level of warmth, as discussed in Chapter 8.

+ **Slips and falls**: Adequate footing must be ensured when traveling over ice. Extra caution must be taken if you must cross frozen water. Ice can be deceptively thin and easily broken through. The depth of snow can also be misleading.

+ **Terrain**: The U.S. *Army Tactics, Techniques, and Procedures: Cold Region Operations* manual recommends travel on major road networks to reduce the potential hidden dangers in snow and ice.

+ **Sunburn**: The sun's rays reflecting off the snow can cause sunburn on exposed skin. Apply sunscreen lotion and protective lip balm, as detailed in the guidelines starting on page 70.

+ **Snow blindness**: Wear sunglasses or cut slits in a piece of cardboard to see through to avoid the dangerous ultraviolet rays of the sun reflecting off the snow.

One of the sneakiest dangers in polar regions is dehydration. Most people are not aware of how much they sweat in cold weather because it's wicked away under multiple layers of clothing. You also lose moisture in your body every time you exhale. It is recommended to consume a gallon and a half of water per day per person to avoid dehydration and maintain normal body function in polar regions. Watch for the symptoms of dehydration: dry mouth, dizziness, cramps, and weakness, among other things. If you begin to see signs of dehydration, treat immediately (see page 72).

To greatly reduce your risk of medical issues in a dangerously cold climate, take steps to ensure you are hydrated. Protect your core temperature and skin by dressing in layers and wearing sunscreen. Secure shelter as soon as possible to begin protecting any lifesaving warmth that you can generate.

FIRE IN COLD ENVIRONMENTS

Believe it or not, fire is not necessarily your first priority in cold-weather climates. Adequate clothing and shelter come first. Because your body creates its own heat, being able to retain that heat may be enough to sustain you until you can save yourself or be saved. Finding items that will burn in a frozen environment may be extremely difficult. Dead trees and, if you have the ability to obtain it, blubber are both flammable options. Because animal blubber may be difficult to procure unless you are familiar with how to do so, you should know how to locate wood in polar climates.

Certain trees are more conducive to burning than others. For example, spruce and birch trees have qualities that may be useful when looking for fuel to burn. Spruce makes excellent firewood and will burn virtually smoke-free in the fall and winter, and the bark of birch trees makes excellent tinder (as do dry, dead leaves and pine needles). First look for dead trees. They will most readily burn, and it can be easier to break their branches into small, usable pieces of firewood. While bark can be good for fire tinder, usually the best firewoods will be bare of bark.

Fuels in polar climates:

+ Dead tree branches

+ Dead grasses tied in bundles

+ Dry animal dung

+ Peat moss (often found in bogs)

When you build a fire in the snow, you're going to need a dry base. A fire built directly on snow or ice will cause melting, and the resulting water can extinguish the fire. Locate a piece of dry ground, a flat rock, or even a base of green logs to build your fire on. Gather enough tinder to give the fire a strong head start. Many survival experts recommend gathering enough tinder and firewood for three fires. That way you'll have plenty once the fire gets going and will hopefully avoid the need to go out and gather more. Block your fire from the wind and be aware of carbon monoxide.

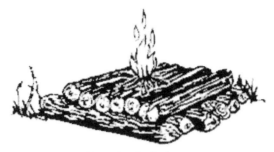

Example of a fire base

Carbon monoxide (CO) is a byproduct of combustion. Any flame will give off a certain amount of CO. It is an extremely insidious chemical, being tasteless, colorless, and odorless. To avoid being poisoned by carbon monoxide, make sure your fire is in a well-ventilated area. If it is outside, there won't be a ventilation issue, but if you fire is built in a shelter, ensure you have adequate ventilation that will allow the CO to escape. The military technical bulletin *Prevention and Management of Cold-Weather Injuries* states very clearly not to sleep in an enclosed area where an open fire is burning.

If you have sand and rocks available, it's a good idea to utilize them. Build a small fire on a pound or so of sand. The heated sand can be used to dry boots and clothing, and you can place it in a small, safe container to be kept in your pocket as a hand warmer. Heated rocks can do the same, and can also be brought into your shelter to safely provide a heat source.

WATER IN COLD ENVIRONMENTS

There are many sources of water in arctic and subarctic regions. Water sources in these area are more sanitary than those in other types of regions due to the climatic and environmental conditions. However, you should still always purify the water before drinking it.

Your location and the season of the year will determine where and how you obtain water. During the summer months, the best natural sources of water are freshwater lakes, streams, ponds, rivers, and springs. Water from ponds or lakes may be slightly stagnant, but still usable. Running water in streams, rivers, and bubbling springs is usually fresh and suitable for drinking. The brownish surface water found in a tundra during the summer is also a good source of water. However, you may have to filter the water before purifying it (see page 133).

You can melt freshwater ice and snow for water. Only use snow if it is bright white and untainted, not touched or discolored in any way. If you have trouble finding snow like this, you can dig below the surface to find clean snow. Completely melt both snow and ice before putting them in your mouth. Trying to melt these in your mouth lowers your core body temperature and may cause internal cold injuries. You can use body heat to melt snow. Place the snow in a water bag and place the bag between your layers of clothing. This is a slow process, but you can use it on the move or when you have no fire.

Fresh sea ice is a viable option when it is available. It may taste salty, but if it has been frozen for more than a year, it has lost its salt through leaching and can be melted down for drinking water. You can identify this ice by its bluish color and rounded edges.

Note: Do not waste fuel to melt ice or snow when drinkable water is available from other sources.

When ice is available, melt it rather than snow. One cup of ice yields more water than one cup of snow does. Ice also takes less time to melt. You can melt ice or snow in a water bag, MRE ration bag, tin can, or improvised container by placing the container near a fire. Begin with a small amount of ice or snow in the container and, as it turns to water, add more ice or snow. Another way to melt ice or snow is by putting it in a bag made from porous material, such as mesh or even cotton, and suspending the bag near the fire. Place a container under the bag to catch the water. During cold weather, avoid drinking a lot of liquid before going to bed. Crawling out of a warm sleeping bag at night to urinate means less rest and more exposure to the cold. Once you have water, keep it next to you to prevent refreezing. Also, do not fill your canteen or water bottle completely. Allowing the water to slosh around will help keep it from freezing.

Here are a few tips for obtaining water in a cold climate:

+ Melt ice rather than snow when available.

+ Choose freshwater ice rather than saltwater ice.

+ Choose snow that is compact—this has the least air and yields the most water.

+ Melt snow inside a container placed in your clothing (but not in direct contact with skin).

+ Melt snow in a porous container over a collection vessel near a fire.

+ Place snow on a clean, dark surface in sunlight.

+ Don't melt snow in your hand and drink unless absolutely necessary—this could lead to cold injuries to your hand.

COLD ENVIRONMENT SHELTERS

In cold environments, depending on your surroundings and the type of equipment you carry, you can build shelters in wooded areas, open country, or barren areas. Wooded areas are usually the best location, providing timber for shelter construction, wood for fire, concealment from observation, and protection from the wind. Barren areas have only snow as building material. Fortunately, snow has natural insulating properties, which means, in some scenarios, simply digging a snow cave or shaping snow into a shelter.

Note: In extreme cold, do not use metal, such as an aircraft fuselage, for shelter. The metal will conduct away from the shelter what little heat you can generate.

Shelters made from ice or snow usually require tools such as ice axes or saws. You must also expend considerable time and energy to build such a shelter. Expending a lot of energy, especially without the food and water necessary to refuel, can be dangerous. If you choose or are forced to create this type of shelter, pace yourself and conserve energy when you can.

Be sure to ventilate an enclosed shelter, especially if you intend to build a fire in it. Always block a shelter's entrance, if possible, to keep the heat in and the wind out. Use a rucksack or snow block. Construct a shelter no larger than needed. This will reduce the amount of space to heat. A fatal error in cold-weather shelter construction is making the shelter so large that it steals body heat rather than saving it. Keep shelter space small. Never sleep directly on the ground. Lay down some pine boughs, grass, or other insulating material to keep the ground from absorbing your body heat.

There are supplies that you'll want to have to for your cold-climate shelter. In a survival situation, you won't have the opportunity to plan ahead and bring all the necessary gear with you. If you have the opportunity, though, to pack supplies for your shelter, consider these:

+ A compact folding shovel

+ Vinyl tent patches

+ Snow saw or knife

+ A "mummy"-style sleeping bag

+ A pad to place under your sleeping bag

Tent

Other than an actual structure like a hunting lodge or cabin, a tent will be your next best option for shelter in a cold climate. Tents are lightweight, portable, and keep you warm and dry. If you're taking a tent into cold-weather conditions, keep these tips in mind:

+ The tent should not be much larger than the occupant to conserve body heat.

+ Tent poles should be sturdy enough to withstand blizzard conditions.

+ Seams should be sealed with water-based urethane sealer.

+ Treat the tent to make the exterior waterproof.

Snow Cave Shelter

The snow cave shelter is a very effective shelter because of the insulating qualities of snow. Remember that it takes time and energy to build, and that you will get wet while constructing it. When building a snow cave, keep these tips in mind:

+ Find a drift about 10 feet deep into which you can dig.

+ Keep the roof arched for strength and to allow melted snow to drain down the sides.

+ Build a sleeping platform higher than the entrance. Separate the sleeping platform from the snow cave's walls, or dig a small trench

between the platform and the wall. This platform will prevent
the melting snow from getting you and your equipment wet. This
construction is especially important if you have a good source of heat
in the snow cave.

+ Ensure the roof is high enough so that you can sit up on the sleeping
platform.

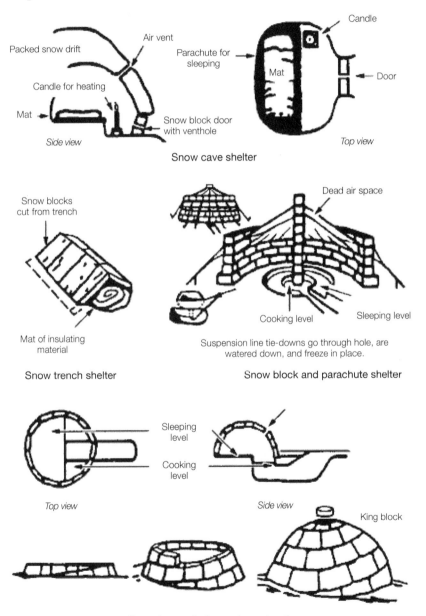

Snow cave shelter

Snow trench shelter

Snow block and parachute shelter

Snow house design and construction

+ Block the entrance with a snow block or other material, and use the lower entrance area for cooking.

+ The walls and ceiling should be at least 12 inches thick.

+ Install a ventilation shaft to allow any carbon monoxide from a heating source or carbon dioxide from your exhalations to vent the snow cave.

+ If you do not have a drift large enough to build a snow cave, you can make a variation of it by piling snow into a mound large enough to dig out.

FOOD IN COLD ENVIRONMENTS

Just as your body requires less food in high-heat conditions, it will require more food in cold-weather conditions—fuel for the furnace, so to speak. You will burn calories simply trying to maintain a normal internal temperature. Starvation is common in extreme cold-weather climates because of the caloric demands on the body. You have to expend energy in order to gather firewood and to build a shelter, and then you need to eat to restore those calories, as well as maintain a healthy core temperature. An adult will burn anywhere from 1,600 to 2,800 calories per day under normal conditions. The same adult should plan on consuming 5,000 calories in a polar region.

Edible Plants in Cold Environments

Although tundras support a variety of plants during the warm months, all those plants are small when compared to those in warmer climates. For instance, the arctic willow and birch are shrubs rather than trees. The following is a list of some plant foods found in arctic and subarctic regions.

+ **Arctic raspberry and blueberry**: Found in the northern landscapes of Alaska, Canada, and other arctic climates, these berries have been eaten as medicine against scurvy and are believed to reduce the chances of developing cardiovascular disease, bronchitis, and urinary tract infections.

+ **Arctic willow**: Located in clumps that cover the tundra, the arctic willow grows to be about 2 feet tall. The outer bark of young shoots can be stripped off and the inner portion eaten raw. The willow leaves can be eaten raw or brewed into a tea for a significant source of vitamin C.

+ **Bearberry**: This is an evergreen shrub that has reddish, scaly bark; thick, leathery leaves; and bright white flowers. The berries can be eaten raw or cooked, and the leaves can be brewed into a tea.

+ **Cranberry**: Growing along the ground with tiny leaves arranged in an alternating pattern along the stem, this plant produces bright red berries that can be eaten raw, though they are very tart. They can be boiled in water to be made more palatable. The berries are used as a diuretic and as treatment for urinary tract infections.

+ **Crowberry**: This is a small evergreen shrub with small, needlelike leaves that grows small, shiny, black berries on it in the winter. These can be eaten straight off the plant.

+ **Dandelion**: These are common throughout North America, easily identified by their bright yellow flowers. All parts of the dandelion are edible. The leaves can be eaten raw or cooked, and the roots can be dried and used as a coffee substitute. Dandelions are high in vitamin A, vitamin C, and calcium.

Dandelion

+ **Eskimo potato**: Also known as the alpine sweetvetch, this plant is commonly found across Alaska and northern Canada. It grows to be 2 inches tall and has light pink or purple flowers emerging on one side of its stalk. Its roots can be eaten raw, steamed, or simmered, and are commonly used in a variety of dishes. Note that while the roots are edible, the seeds are not; they are believed to be toxic. These seeds possibly caused the death of Christopher McCandless, made famous by the book and movie *Into the Wild*.

+ **Iceland moss**: This is gray, white, or reddish moss that grows only a few inches high. All parts of it are edible and can be eaten raw, but boiling it will remove some of the bitterness.

+ **Reindeer moss**: This moss grows to be only a few inches tall and does not flower. Although it has a crunchy, brittle texture, the entire plant is edible. It can be soaked in water to soften and remove some of its bitterness.

+ **Spruce needles**: These are high in vitamin C and commonly brewed as a tea. The type of needle chosen affects the flavor of the tea; light green spruce tips will yield a light, slightly lemony flavor, while mature needles harvested during the winter will create a stronger taste. Rather than boiling the needles directly in water, boil water separately and pour it over the crushed needles in order to retain their nutrients.

Avoid these plants:

+ **Arctic poppy**: poisonous flower

+ **Bearded lichen**: acid causes stomach irritation

+ **Lupine and larkspur**: toxic wildflowers

+ **Water hemlock**: fatal if consumed

Edible Animals in Cold Environments

+ **Fish and fish eggs**: Do not eat fish if they have sunken eyes, are slimy to the touch rather than moist or wet, or have a sharp and foul taste. To prepare a fish, cut along its bottom and remove all the "guts." The *US Army Survival Manual* recommends cooking all freshwater fish. Some saltwater fish can be eaten raw. The head can be removed prior to cooking, but this isn't necessary.

+ **Clams, mussels, and oysters**: Popular opinion states that the "R rule" should be followed when eating clams or mussels. This rule means that they should only be eaten in months that have an "r" in their names. So, clams and mussels are safe to eat from September through April, but should be avoided in summer months due to high concentrations of algae. They should be eaten alive, since they spoil quickly. If a shell is already gaped, you can assume the creature is dead and so should not be eaten. Clams, mussels, and oysters can be baked, boiled, steamed, broiled, grilled, or fried.

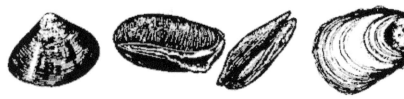

Clams, mussels, and oysters

+ **Sea urchin eggs**: Known as "roe," these are a bright yellow color and can be found inside female sea urchins, which are more reddish-brown than black. The roe can be eaten raw, but they are hard to obtain. Use caution when slicing the spines of sea urchins and cutting into the shell.

+ **Sea cucumber**: These are popular in Asia for their rubbery texture. They can be prepared several ways, but one simple and common method is to clean out their insides, rinse, soak in cold water for at least half a day, and then simmer for several hours.

+ **Owls and ptarmigans**: Owls are difficult to snare since they are nocturnal. Even when caught, they are mostly feathers and do not have much meat. If eating an owl, remove all the feathers and thoroughly cook the meat. A ptarmigan is a small game bird that can be easier to catch than an owl and should be cooked the same way.

+ **Bird eggs**: It is rare for a wild bird to lay an unfertilized egg. If you access a nest, you can expect the eggs to be fertilized, containing a fetus. If the eggs are not fertilized, you can cook them as you would the eggs of a chicken.

+ **Foxes and weasels**: Unless you are trained in making wild animal snares, you will have a difficult time harvesting a fox or weasel. Also keep in mind that foxes are often rabid, and you should never risk eating an animal with rabies. If you are able to kill a fox or weasel and are sure it is healthy, remove the meat and cook it thoroughly.

+ **Deer and caribou**: If you have a firearm capable of taking them down, you may be able to harvest deer or caribou. Otherwise, there is very little chance of catching one. As with other wild meat, you should ensure it is cooked completely before consuming.

+ **Seals and penguins**: You will likely need a firearm and a boat in order to catch one of these creatures. Seals and penguins can be eaten, but should only be hunted if nothing else is available. To eat a penguin, remove all the blubber before cooking the meat. To eat a seal, remove all the blubber and cut it into strips. These will dissolve into oil that can be used for cooking. The meat can be cooked in a variety of ways, including simply boiling.

Avoid these animals:

+ **Black mussels**: toxic

+ **Greenland shark**: toxic

+ **Polar bears**: aggressive and extremely dangerous to humans—found along coastlines where seals are plentiful (rather than inland)

+ **Grizzly bears and gray wolves**: can be aggressive and dangerous, though will usually avoid humans if they can help it

+ **Ravens**: usually don't have enough meat to make it worth the hunt

+ **Sculpin eggs**: toxic

+ **Walruses**: far more dangerous than people expect

+ **Black flies**: bites are painful—avoid them by wearing a mosquito net and by not camping near water where they feed and swarm in late spring and early summer

COLD ENVIRONMENT MEDICINAL PLANTS

Chaga: Also known as "tiaga" and "tsi aga," this plant has been simmered (boiling has been found to decrease its medicinal properties) as tea and used as an anti-inflammatory, natural energy booster, and topical treatment for skin conditions such as psoriasis and eczema, among other things.

Identification:

+ Fungal growth often found on birch trees

+ Usually black, brittle, and cracked

+ Forms within the tree and grows through the bark

Arctic willow: The inner portion and the underground roots can be eaten and used to ease a toothache and on wounds to stop bleeding, and consumed to ease digestive issues.

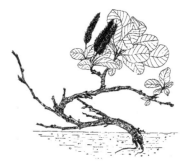

Arctic willow

Identification:

+ Typically grow only to about 6 inches (can be much larger in the Pacific Northwest)

+ Round, shiny green leaves about 1½ inches long

+ Dioecious (having male and female parts)—male plants have yellow flowering spikes and females have red

Labrador tea: The leaves are simmered to be consumed as a tea for a sore throat, cough, or chest congestion. Labrador tea has also been used to treat diarrhea, muscle pains, and headaches.

Identification:

+ Grows to 4 to 5 feet tall

+ Will grow straight up in southern latitudes, but in arctic regions will grow as ground cover

+ Woolly branches

+ Narrow 1- to 2-inch leaves

+ Tiny clusters of white flowers

Bearberry: A common evergreen shrub whose leaves can be brewed as a tea, or its berries can be eaten cooked or raw. Bearberry is a diuretic that helps remove excess fluids from the body through urine, and is also a strong astringent that contracts tissue and can reduce inflammation and bleeding.

Identification:

+ Shrub

+ Reddish, scaly bark

+ Thick, leathery leaves

+ White flowers

+ Bright red berries

Sweet cicely: A bushy perennial, the entire sweet cicely plant can be consumed. The leaves can be eaten raw or cooked to treat coughs, upset stomach, and flatulence. The root is antiseptic and has been used to treat bites and wounds

Identification:

+ 1½ to 3 inches tall

+ Light green, lacy leaves

+ Delicate white flowers

+ Long, pointed seeds

MOUNTAINS

Mountains are one of the most treacherous environments in which to travel and survive. Your physical condition is top priority in these regions. It takes great strength and stamina to navigate your way around, as well as a good level of cardiovascular fitness. Simply traversing the rocks, cliffs, trees, and trenches can be too much for many people. When you factor in the altitude, it adds an entire new degree of challenge. The air is thin at higher elevations, making it difficult to breathe. Most experts will tell you to allow yourself 7 to 10 days to acclimate your body to the altitude before exerting yourself. In a survival situation, you don't always have that option.

The U.S. military technical bulletin *Altitude Acclimatization and Illness Management* states, "Within the U.S., few military installations are located at altitude. Even at these installations, the area available for maneuvers may be very limited. Nevertheless, the lack of familiarity and experience with strategies to cope with this unique environment should not be minimized because altitude exposure can deleteriously affect health, mental and physical performance, and morale."

To achieve maximum physical performance in higher altitudes, certain physiological changes known as "acclimatization" must occur. Your body must adapt to the lower oxygen saturation found at higher elevations. As you ascend or descend, your body will acclimate to your new altitude, but it will require time to do so. Changing elevations too rapidly can cause altitude sickness (see page 172).

Four factors affect acclimatization in mountainous terrain:

+ Altitude

+ Rate of ascent

+ Duration of stay

+ Level of exertion

Like a scuba diver descending and ascending in water, someone climbing to higher altitudes must factor in all of the above. Adjustments in altitude must be paced and staged.

High altitude causes certain symptoms that are typical responses of acclimating bodies, not indications of altitude illness. Normal responses to high altitude:

+ Hyperventilation

+ Difficult and labored breathing during exertion (*not* when resting)

+ Increased urination

+ Awakening many times at night, sometimes to urinate

+ Periodic breathing at night

+ Swelling of the face and feet

Periodic breathing is when someone, while sleeping, stops breathing for no more than 10 seconds and then has a series of rapid, shallow breaths. It is not a sign of altitude sickness; it occurs in everyone above their personal altitude threshold. It may disturb sleep. The swelling of the face and feet is a symptom more common for women than for men. None of these symptoms require you to descend to lower altitudes.

MOUNTAIN HAZARDS

Mountainous regions can feature a multitude of climates, and thus a multitude of hazards. In any case, you can best ensure safety and survival by taking certain preventative measures. Procuring food and water is vital and will be discussed later in this chapter. In the mountains, beyond basic survival needs, you should be aware of the terrain, dangerous animals, and the weather. Steep drop-offs can be instantly deadly, loose rocks or mud have the potential to create a dangerous scenario, and snow and thunderstorms are particularly violent in the mountains. Wildlife, while abundant and possibly providing you the nutritional sustenance to survive, can also be deadly. Bites, stings, and attacks are possible from dozens of living things all around you in the mountains.

It is critically important to be ever-vigilant when in the mountains. Seek shelter early and be keenly aware of your surroundings and weather. Treat medical issues as soon as they arise according to the steps outlined in the appropriate chapter in this book. The following are some of the most common medical issues that occur in the mountains.

+ **Falls**: Be aware of your surroundings and vigilant in ensuring your footing.

+ **Fractures**: Uneven mountainous terrain leads to fractures. Treat as outlined in Chapter 5.

+ **Lacerations**: Scrapes and cuts are common and should be treated according to the bleeding control steps in Chapter 2.

+ **Bites and stings**: Treat according to Chapter 10.

+ **Temperature-related illnesses**: Even mild temperatures can lead to hot- or cold-related illnesses. See Chapter 7 for heat emergencies and Chapter 8 for cold emergencies.

The primary hazards in the mountains come in the forms of altitude illnesses, avalanches, and weather. You should also be aware of a number of animal hazards.

Altitude Illnesses

The *US Marine Corps Summer Survival Course Handbook* warns us that even highly fit, motivated individuals may become victims of altitude sickness or much more serious conditions. Some people are just more susceptible to high altitudes than others, and the reason why is not known. For example, two sisters I know went backpacking in the Sierras. They were almost exactly the same height and weight, and were only five years apart in age. On reaching 11,000 feet, the older sister became very ill and started to black out while the younger sister felt fine. If you find yourself strongly affected by high altitudes, this does not mean you are weak or out of shape. Listen to your body and take a break. Slow and easy climbing, limited activity, and long rest periods are critical to altitude acclimatization and survival.

Acute mountain sickness (AMS): This is what we know as altitude sickness. It is common with rapid ascent over 8,000 feet, though it can occur at lower altitudes. It is fairly common, experienced by 6.5 percent of men and 22.2 percent of women at 7,800 to 1,500 feet. At higher altitudes, such as 13,800 feet, 80 percent of people experience AMS. It can begin anywhere from 8 to 96 hours after reaching a high altitude. The brain undergoes very minor swelling, resulting in the following symptoms.

Signs and Symptoms

+ Throbbing headache on the sides or back of head that gets worse when bending over

+ Loss of appetite

+ Nausea or vomiting

+ Sleep disturbance

+ Fatigue

+ Dizziness

Treatment

Since many AMS symptoms are the same as those experienced with dehydration, the first course of treatment should be giving the patient water. If they improve, then they probably do not have AMS and are just dehydrated. If they do have AMS, there are a few things that can be done to mitigate the effects:

+ Climb high, sleep low. Limit the altitude at which you sleep to no more than a 1,000 feet increase per day.

+ Avoid alcohol and sedatives.

+ Moderate exertion helps. Too much exertion just makes it worse.

+ If immediate treatment is desired, descend 3,000 feet.

+ To acclimatize, rest at the same elevation at least one hour and up to 48 hours. If prescribed, take acetazolamide (Diamox) to cut down the resting time to 12 to 24 hours. Dexamethasone (Decadron) cuts down the resting time to an even shorter 2 to 6 hours. If given oxygen or hyperbaric treatment, you only need to rest for 2 hours.

+ It is possible that gingko helps with AMS, though studies are inconclusive.

+ As odd as it may sound, Viagra and other erectile dysfunction (ED) medications help some people at high altitude.

Prevention

If you know you are susceptible to AMS, see if your doctor will prescribe you dexamethasone or acetazolamide. These can be taken for a few days before you ascend as a preventative measure.

High-altitude cerebral edema (HACE): This is a severe form of AMS in which the brain swells even more. Patients will always experience AMS before HACE, but denial of AMS is very common. HACE is very rare below 14,000 feet, though it does occur in 1 percent of people above 8,800 feet. If not treated, HACE can lead to delirium, coma, and death.

Signs and Symptoms

Those with HACE experience all the same signs and symptoms as AMS, in addition to:

+ **Gait ataxia**: lack of control of muscle movement, bad coordination, sometimes an odd walk

+ **Mental status**: brain doesn't function as well, slow and easily confused

Treatment

Immediate treatment of HACE is vital. It is a medical emergency, and deaths have occurred at only 11,500 feet. Within hours, the patient will go into a coma. There are a few ways to treat HACE:

+ *Go down*. The importance of descending cannot be emphasized enough. This is the only certain treatment for HACE.

+ Take dexamethasone.

+ Receive an oxygen treatment.

+ Receive hyperbaric treatment—this requires a total body chamber that has controllable atmospheric pressure and 100 percent oxygen.

High-altitude pulmonary edema (HAPE): This is another altitude illness, but it is different from AMS and HACE. While those illnesses affect the brain, HAPE affects the lungs. It is caused by vascular leaks in the lungs, high blood pressure, and swelling in the lungs. It can be fatal.

Signs and Symptoms

Patients with HAPE will experience at least two of the following:

+ Difficult and labored breathing when resting

+ Abnormally rapid breathing or heart rate

+ Crackles or wheezing in breathing

+ A cough, sometimes producing a pink, frothy substance

+ Chest tightness or congestion

+ Decreased exercise tolerance or severe fatigue

+ Bluish discoloration of skin

+ Fever

Treatment

As with HACE, HAPE is a medical emergency. Failure to descend will result in death in a few hours. HAPE has a 10 to 15 percent mortality rate even with treatment.

+ *Go down*. You must immediately descend. Cold temperatures increase the swelling of the lungs, so patients may be too weak to walk. If this is the case, carry or drag them down.

+ Receive an oxygen treatment.

+ Use a Gamow bag, often present at aid stations in the mountains. It is an inflatable pressure bag big enough to fit a person inside, and simulates the conditions at lower altitudes.

Avalanche

An avalanche can occur in nearly any type of weather and quickly destroys everything in its path. Avalanches occur when stress is added to a slope. The stress can come from snow, rain, falling rocks, temperature changes, or simply the weight of a human or animal. Most occur on slopes from 30 to 45 degrees. Because of the difficulty of predicting an avalanche, your best defense could be to simply be aware of your surroundings and what you should do if caught in one. Snow avalanches are survivable if you know these survival tips:

+ Shout to others—if there are people around, they may be able to identify your location after the avalanche occurs.

+ Breathe through your nose.

+ Use a backstroke motion to stay on top of the snow.

+ Thrust an arm upward. Even exposed fingertips can lead to a rescue.

+ Curve your other arm in front of your face and chest to create an air pocket.

+ Stay calm.

+ Keep shouting until rescuers can locate you.

You may not be able to avoid an avalanche, but there are a few steps you can take when traveling through an avalanche zone to reduce your chances of starting one or being caught in one. First and foremost, simply avoid the area if at all possible. Some signs of an avalanche path are broken trees and a chute-like clearing with debris at the bottom. If you can't avoid it, send one person through at a time, thus reducing exposure to the whole group. Before noon, travel in the shade. Rising air temperatures can be the cause of an avalanche. Also, it helps to carry brightly colored avalanche tape, a locator beacon, and a shovel.

Weather

The weather on mountains is varied, it comes in swiftly, and it packs a punch. You often get little or no warning of an oncoming storm that could bring a deluge, lightning strikes, and the potential for mudslides and avalanches. "Sudden" and "potentially fierce" are the best ways to describe weather in the mountains. The wind strikes the mountains differently than other landscapes, which causes inconsistent patterns and localized wind gusts and paths. Storms are channeled by the mountain peaks and rain can set in for hours or even days. Because of the terrain, you don't often have the opportunity to see incoming weather. Mother Nature, however, does offer certain cues that will clue you in to oncoming weather:

+ A halo around the sun or moon can be indicative of a coming storm.

+ Horsetail cirrus clouds thicken and descend when a storm is approaching.

+ Lowering clouds can be indicative of cumulonimbus thunderclouds forming.

+ Rapid wind or temperature changes can also be an indication of an impending weather change.

Thunderstorms are chaotic in the mountains. Numerous lightning strikes, driving rain, and hail frequently lash out against the terrain. Afternoons are the most common times for thunderstorms to strike. If you see evidence of an approaching thunderstorm, avoid ridges and peaks, and get to as low an elevation as possible. Once lightning begins to strike or the storm sets in, seek immediate shelter. Avoid water, metal, and lone trees, which are prone to lightning strikes. Once you've found a sheltered spot, remain there until the storm has passed.

Another less menacing but equally dangerous weather event is fog. When mist and fog set in, you can become disoriented and travel in the wrong direction or even walk right into a deadly scenario or off a cliff. Because of the terrain and changing air masses in the mountains, fog occurs frequently, more commonly on the windward side. Downward-moving layers of stratus clouds trap cold air in the valleys, creating mist. Fog and mist can create a dangerous situation for anyone on the move. Your best option is to wait until it lifts, allowing you to regain your visibility over the terrain and for dangerous wildlife.

Animals

Animal hazards are plentiful in the mountains. Insects can bite and sting, snakes can strike, and bears can attack with little warning. The good news is that the majority of animals are not aggressive. If you're careful and knowledgeable, you can avoid most dangerous encounters. Start by making noise. One of the most dangerous situations you can find yourself in is startling an animal in the mountains. It will likely lash out at you in response to fear.

If you do find yourself in a situation where you have startled a large animal, avoid the urge to turn and run. That urge will be *very* strong, but if you give in to it, the animal will view you as prey and instinctively chase. Instead, back away slowly until you are safe. If you are unable to successfully back away, you may try shouting at them.

Avoid these animals:

+ **Grizzly bear**: Do not turn and run. If possible, back away slowly. Bears have poor eyesight and may not recognize you as human if you get far enough away. If it attacks you, lie face down and play dead. If it rolls you over, continue to roll until you are face down. Attack the bear only as a last resort.

+ **Black bear**: Do not play dead. Back away slowly if you can. Bears have poor eyesight and may not recognize you as human if you get far enough away. Fight with sticks, rocks, or anything else you have available to you. Do not try running or climbing to evade it because it is faster and a better climber than you.

+ **Rattlesnake**: Use caution with where you put your hands and feet. If you hear the telltale rattle, back away slowly. In case of a snakebite, follow the procedures outlined on page 105.

+ **Scorpions**: Scorpions come out at night. Shake out clothing and boots before putting them on. Scorpion stings are rarely fatal. In case of a scorpion sting, follow the procedures outlined on page 99.

+ **Cougar (mountain lion)**: Do not turn and run. Attempt to make yourself look larger by raising your hands and spreading out your jacket. Make noise and throw things but do not bend over to pick anything up, thus appearing smaller and more vulnerable.

+ **Moose**: Moose are aggressive. If you encounter one, back away slowly and change direction.

FIRE IN THE MOUNTAINS

The majority of mountainous climates, unless snow-covered, are rich in fuels for building a fire. Fallen trees, dead grasses, and shrubbery abound in the foothills and angular formations that climb toward the peaks. It is only at a certain height that the air becomes too thin to sustain most plant life. Known as the "tree line," this is a clear line on mountains where trees no longer grow.

The height of the tree line varies depending on many factors. For example, in Colorado it's at approximately 12,000 feet. By contrast, it's at around 2,000 feet in Scotland. Above the tree line, only limited vegetation grows, so locating fire fuel can become more difficult. Your best fuel sources above the tree line will be scrub brush and stunted trees.

You must be careful building a fire in the mountains. A fire should be made on bare dirt or rock and well away from combustible materials—a fire can quickly get out of control and lead to unimaginable devastation. There are additional hazards when creating a fire in the mountains such as high winds, rain or snow, and lightning. You can build a trench or place stacked rocks in a semicircular pattern around the fire to protect the fire from the elements and the topography from the fire.

If you need to build a fire after rainfall or snow, there are some steps you can take to possibly utilize wet wood.

1. Gather some kindling (dry dead leaves, scrub brush, or dead wood that is about as wide as your finger or less).

2. Use a knife or hatchet to strip away as much bark and outer layers of the wet wood as possible.

3. Split larger pieces of wood into kindling, exposing the drier inner layers.

4. Start a small fire using the kindling.

5. Use the small fire to heat and dry the larger pieces. There will likely be a lot of steam and smoke, but it should subside after a few minutes.

WATER IN THE MOUNTAINS

At higher elevations the body loses considerable amounts of water due to a combination of perspiration, urination, and rapid breathing. The amount of water you will need to consume is dependent on your level of exertion. As a general rule, an individual should consume 4 to 8 quarts of water a day in low mountains and may need 10 or more quarts of water at higher elevations. Thirst and sweat are not good indicators of fluid loss. By the time a person feels thirsty, they are already dehydrated. Sweat is absorbed in clothing and evaporates too rapidly to typically be noticed. You should make every attempt to be one step ahead of dehydration by consuming a healthy amount of water or other decaffeinated fluids.

The *US Army Survival Manual* states:

> *When soldiers become thirsty, they are already dehydrated. Loss of body water also plays a major role in causing altitude sickness and cold injury. Forced drinking in the absence of thirst, monitoring the deepness of the yellow hue in the urine, and watching for behavioral symptoms common to altitude sickness are important factors for commanders to consider in assessing the water balance of soldiers operating in the mountains.*

Military survival guides say that in the mountains, as elsewhere, refilling each soldier's water container as often as possible is mandatory. No matter how pure and clean mountain water may appear, water from natural sources should always be purified or chemically sterilized to prevent parasitic illnesses (giardiasis). Commanders should consider requiring the increased use of individual packages of powdered drink mixes, fruit, and juices to help encourage the required fluid intake. The same rules apply to anyone who finds themselves traveling or fighting for survival in the mountains.

The best natural sources of water are freshwater lakes, streams, ponds, rivers, and springs. Water from ponds or lakes may be slightly stagnant, but still usable. Running water in streams, rivers, and bubbling springs is usually fresh and suitable for drinking, though it should still be purified if possible. If these large bodies of water are not around, there are other, less obvious sources of water in the mountains.

Hidden natural water sources include:

+ Porous limestone encourages seepage—look for rocky ground.

+ Clay bluffs hold water—look for green vegetation indicating its presence.

+ Cliff bases may contain collected runoff water.

+ Dry streambeds—water may be just below the surface.

MOUNTAIN SHELTERS

Mountains can provide a vast array of weather even in a single day. Heat, rain, wind, lightning, and snow can all potentially occur depending on the mountain, the elevation, and the time of year. Even in the warmest climates, there can be snow at higher altitudes. In most mountain regions there are abundant natural shelters that you can utilize for warmth and to stay safe and dry. The U.S. Marine Corps survival manual also gives several options for man-made shelters, including stone circle and rock outcropping shelters.

Stone Circle Shelter

If you find yourself in an area where you have access to a lot of stones, you can use them to your advantage by building a stone circle shelter.

1. Without being in an avalanche or flood area, locate a depression in the ground.

2. Use the stones to build a low wall around the depression.

3. Do not make it too big—it will be difficult to heat or possibly collapse.

4. Cover the space with branches and then foliage to provide insulation.

5. Fill the gaps in the stones with mud to provide additional insulation.

Rock Outcropping Shelter

1. Anchor one end of your poncho, canvas, parachute, or other material on the edge of the outcropping using rocks or other weights.

2. Extend and anchor the other end of the material so it provides the best possible shade.

FOOD IN THE MOUNTAINS

Caloric intake is extremely important at higher altitudes. Your level of exertion is greatly increased, and it's possible for a single person to burn 15,000 calories in one day. Soldiers and outdoor adventurers carry with them meals and snacks that are high in carbohydrates and calories. There are plentiful options for natural food found in the wilderness of the mountains, but packing your own food, if that is an option, is the easiest and safest means to provide food in a mountainous climate.

Poor nutrition contributes to illness or injury, decreased performance, poor morale, and susceptibility to cold injuries, and can severely affect military operations. Influences at high altitudes that can affect nutrition include a dulled taste sensation (making food undesirable), nausea, and lack of energy or motivation to prepare or eat meals. Caloric requirements increase in the mountains due to both the altitude and the cold. A diet high in fat and carbohydrates is important in helping the body fight the effects of these conditions. Fats provide long-term, slow caloric release, but are often unpalatable to people who are experiencing the ill effects of operating at higher altitudes.

Products that can seriously impact performance in mountainous terrain include:

+ **Tobacco**: Tobacco smoke interferes with oxygen delivery by reducing the blood's oxygen-carrying capacity. Tobacco smoke in close, confined spaces increases the amounts of carbon monoxide. The irritant effect of tobacco smoke may produce a narrowing of airways, interfering with optimal air movement. Smoking can effectively raise the "physiological altitude" by as much as several hundred meters.

+ **Alcohol**: Alcohol impairs judgment and perception, depresses respiration, causes dehydration, and increases susceptibility to cold injury.

+ **Caffeine**: Caffeine may improve physical and mental performance, but it also causes increased urination (leading to dehydration), and therefore should be consumed in moderation.

Above the tree line, options for food are scarce. At lower elevations, below the tree line, plant and wildlife food options are plentiful. Plants and animals should only be consumed in a survival situation. A good idea would be to have a guidebook for your region showing all of the edible plants that includes pictures and the best ways to consume them. You should be extremely careful before eating plants unless you can positively identify them and are certain it is safe to do so. Choosing the wrong plant could have dire consequences. Berries, for example, are bright colored and can be extremely inviting, but can be either delicious and nutritious, or, at the other extreme, toxic and deadly.

Edible Mountainous Plants

+ **Lichens**: These must be soaked overnight and then boiled.

+ **Balsam root**: This root can be eaten raw or cooked.

+ **Spruce needles**: Boil them for a boost of vitamin C.

+ **Birch tree**: Both the tree's sap and inner bark can be eaten raw or boiled.

+ **Piñon nuts**: These can be eaten raw or roasted.

+ **Young pine cones**: These can be boiled or baked.

+ **Juniper berries**: These berries can be eaten raw or cooked.

+ **Dandelions**: One of the most common weeds found in North America, dandelions are not only the bane of groundskeepers, but also are entirely edible, are high in vitamin A and C and even calcium, and can be eaten in a variety of ways. The flowers, leaves, and buds can be eaten as a salad, and the roots can be boiled and eaten as well.

Avoid these plants:

+ **Any part of a cedar tree**: Cedar oil can be toxic to humans and animals.

+ **Corn lily (false hellebore)**: This is poisonous to humans.

+ **Death camas (death lily)**: All parts of this plant are toxic and should not be consumed.

+ **Mountain laurel**: This plant is poisonous to humans and animals, so much so that you should wash your hands after handling it to avoid cross contamination.

Mountain laurel

+ **Poison ivy/poison oak**: Their oil is poisonous, causing an allergic reaction on most people's skin when touched. Can be deadly if directly ingested or if they are burned and one breathes in the smoke, so *never* use them as fuel. Poison oak looks deceptively similar to berry bushes, so there is a simple and silly rhyme to help remember the difference:
  Leaves of three, let it be
  If it's hairy, it's a berry
  If it's shiny, watch your heinie.

Edible Mountainous Animals

Wildlife provides another food option if you have the ability to kill it. Mountainous regions provide a wide range of edible options.

+ **Deer and elk**: These are plentiful, but can be difficult to kill without a firearm.

+ **Mountain goats**: These are also abundant, but like deer and elk, can be challenging to harvest.

+ **Rabbits**: Rabbits are smaller and far easier to catch, but unfortunately don't provide much nutritional value and may not be worth the effort required to catch them.

+ **Fish**: Fish seem to provide the most bang for your buck. Anywhere there's water, you're likely to find fish. Learn how to fashion a makeshift line and hook or other means to catch fish in the wilderness without fishing gear. This skill alone could mean the difference between life and death.

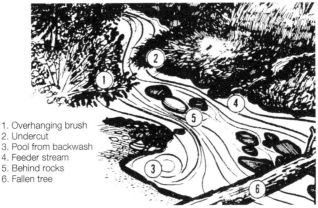

1. Overhanging brush
2. Undercut
3. Pool from backwash
4. Feeder stream
5. Behind rocks
6. Fallen tree

Places where fish tend to gather

MOUNTAINOUS MEDICINAL PLANTS

Navajo tea: Navajo tea is known as Cota and Greenthread, among other names, and is typically found at elevations above 4,500 feet. Navajo tea has been used for centuries to treat urinary tract infections (UTIs); it can also treat an upset stomach, and can even be used as a stimulant. The leaves can be brewed along with the flowers for a slightly sweeter taste.

Identification:

+ Radiant yellow flower

+ Flowers are often ½ to 1 inch in size

+ Long slender stalks

+ Leaves grow opposite each other along the stalk

White horsemint: This has a variety of uses, including brewing the leaves in a tea to treat nausea, indigestion, and vomiting. It can also lessen the pain of arthritis by increasing blood flow through the area and hastening the removal of toxins. White horsemint is also a rich source of the antiseptic thymol, which is sometimes used in mouthwash and toothpaste.

Identification:

+ 1 to 4 feet tall

+ Strongly aromatic

+ Downy leaves dotted with small depressions

+ Oval to triangular 5-inch leaves

+ Two lipped flowers

+ Pale blue, white, rose, or violet flowers

Skullcap: This is a powerful medicinal herb used to treat a variety of ailments including mental conditions and nervous disorders. It has been successfully utilized in the treatment of ADD, anxiety, and epilepsy. It also has anti-inflammatory and sedative properties, helping to treat insomnia.

Identification:

+ 6 to 18 inches tall

+ Square, hairy stems

+ Heart-shaped leaves opposite each other on the stem

+ ½- to 2½-inch leaves

+ Blue to lavender flowers

Osha root: Native to the mountains of the western United States, this root has a long history of uses by Native Americans that continue to this day, including chewing or brewing the roots into a tea to treat cough, cold, bronchial pneumonia, sore throat, fever, diarrhea, and other gastrointestinal disorders.

Identification:

+ 2 to 4 feet tall

+ Deeply incised elliptic-shaped leaf segments

+ ½- to 1½-inch leaves

+ White, five-petal flowers that appear in late summer

+ In winter the aboveground part dies back to a thick, woody rootstock

Comfrey: Although comfrey actually contains poisonous chemicals, the root, stem, and leaves have medicinal properties. Comfrey is widely used to treat upset stomach, ulcers, diarrhea, heavy menstruation; gargled to treat gum disease and sore throat; and used topically on skin to treat wounds. The leaves can be brewed in a tea and consumed. Externally the tea can be used as a wash, or the crushed root can be directly applied to a wound or burn to help the pain relief and healing process. *Do not* use it on an open wound. Doing so could possibly allow large amounts of the dangerous chemicals in comfrey to enter the bloodstream.

Identification:

+ 2 to 5 feet tall

+ Black, turnip-like root

+ Hairy, broad leaves

+ Bell-shaped flowers of green or purplish color

FORESTS

The forests of America are one of the most popular climates for people looking to get away find themselves. We go fishing, camping, and hiking, and immerse ourselves in the tree-canopied forests that lie beyond the reach of the housing developments. Because of the number of people who wander into the forests, they're also places where thousands of people find themselves lost each year. In most cases, people who get lost know they are not far from civilization and it does not often become a life-and-death ordeal—but it can. As stated throughout the *US Army Survival Manual*, the forest offers a plethora of useful natural resources that can aid you in a survival situation.

The challenges that face people in the forest vary, but are similar to those found in other climates. Weather, terrain, and wildlife can all become adversaries, but can also offer lifesaving water, shelter, and food. It all depends on your ability to recognize the degree of peril you're in and take the appropriate steps to ensure your survival. One also must acknowledge the dynamics of a forest. For example, you may cross a stream heading one direction, and following a rainstorm or if you've been gone for a fair length of time, you may return to find the stream you crossed has become an impassible roaring river.

FOREST HAZARDS

Nearly everything in a forest has the potential to help you in a survival situation. Conversely, nearly everything in a forest has the potential to cause injury or death. Being aware of your surroundings and how to utilize the forest to help you can be the difference between life and death. There are certain injuries that are common in a forest environment that you should expect and be prepared to treat.

+ **Fractures**: Be able to utilize elements of the forest to treat a fracture, as discussed in Chapter 5.

+ **Lacerations**: Control bleeding by following the steps in Chapter 2.

+ **Bites and stings**: Treat according to the steps in Chapter 10.

+ **Temperature-related illnesses**: Even mild temperatures can lead to hot- or cold-related illnesses. See Chapter 7 for heat emergencies and Chapter 8 for cold emergencies.

As with other climates, the best way to prevent injury and illness in a forest is to be diligent in maintaining situational awareness. The terrain, wildlife, and weather are all factors that require constant evaluation. As injuries arise, treat them immediately. Waiting to treat an injury could create further problems, only compounding your peril.

Travel

In a forest climate one of your primary concerns will be travel, particularly in a dense forest where your immediate scenery doesn't seem to change as you progress through the trees. Military survival manuals recommend that to move easily, you must develop "jungle eye"—that is, you should not concentrate on the pattern of bushes and trees to your immediate front. You must focus on the scenery further out and find natural breaks in the foliage. Look *through* the forest, not at it. Stop and stoop down occasionally to look along the forest floor. This may reveal game trails that you can follow. Stay alert and move slowly and steadily through dense forest or jungle. Stop periodically to listen and take your bearings.

Use a machete to cut through dense vegetation, but do not cut unnecessarily or you will quickly wear yourself out. If using a machete, stroke upward when cutting vines to reduce noise, because sound carries long distances in the jungle. Use a stick to part the vegetation. Using a stick will also help dislodge biting ants, spiders, or snakes. *Do not* grasp at brush or vines when climbing slopes; they may have irritating spines or sharp thorns.

Many jungle and forest animals follow game trails. These trails wind and cross, but frequently lead to water or clearings. Use them if they lead in your desired direction of travel. In many countries, electric and telephone lines run for miles through sparsely inhabited areas. Usually, the right-of-way is clear enough to allow easy travel.

Animals

A primary hazard in the forest environment will come in the form of animals. Large animals such as bears can create problems for you and your survival. Your best defense against large animals is avoidance. If you have the opportunity to avoid them, you should! If you do, however, encounter a large animal, you should know what you are up against.

Grizzly bears:

+ Generally solitary animals but can be found in groups near a food source.

+ Are stealthy and will usually only attack when threatened or provoked.

+ Will flatten their ears like a dog when they are about to attack.

+ Respond to an attack by playing dead: Lie face down with your legs spread and your hands on the back of your neck with fingers interlaced.

+ If you end up on your back, roll over onto your stomach.

+ DO NOT attempt to run away.

+ DO NOT attempt to fight back unless the grizzly begins to lick your wounds—this is a sign it is about to eat.

Black bears:

+ Most common bear found in North America.

+ Despite their name, can be a variety of colors.

+ Are also solitary animals.

+ Inquisitive.

+ Unlikely to break off an attack once it has started.

+ Will not stop an attack if you play dead—you must fight back.

+ Try hitting the snout or eyes with your fist, a rock, or a stick.

Tips to avoid a bear attack:

+ When traveling, make noise—don't surprise a bear.

+ Never store food in your tent.

+ Hang food in a bag with a rope thrown over a high tree limb.

+ Bears are more active at dawn and dusk, so plan travel accordingly.

+ Eliminate food odors by removing clothes you wore to cook before going to bed.

+ Be aware that dogs tend to antagonize bears and could provoke an attack.

A bear encounter may be the most frightening scenario you could image in the wilderness, but they are rare. A far more likely situation comes in a much smaller, more silent form. The bite or sting from spiders, mosquitoes, ticks, snakes, and even bees can quickly escalate into a serious medical situation. Every year more people die of anaphylaxis from a bee sting than from snakebites. Particularly if you have an allergy to bee stings, use extra-special caution to avoid being stung. If bites or stings do occur, consult the treatment steps in Chapter 10.

FIRES IN FORESTS

A forest will provide one of the easiest environments in which to locate fuel for starting a fire, typically in the form of tree branches and limbs, dead leaves, and dry shrubbery. Unless there has been significant rainfall, you should be able to locate a plethora of dry fuel to burn. Because logs and branches on the ground tend to absorb moisture from the soil, your best bet is to locate dead sticks and branches that are still attached to a tree. They tend to be drier, even in wet weather.

WATER IN FORESTS

Since forests are typically full of wildlife, paying attention to the animals is a particularly good method of locating water when in a forest environment. Animals need water just as humans do, so if you use your eyes and ears, the local wildlife may lead you to water. At night a good method is to listen for frogs. They gather around water sources and often make enough noise that you can hear it from long distances away. Larger grazing animals also need water, so pay attention to tracks. If you see a convergence of tracks in the dirt, you may be on the right path to a water source.

Water in forests that is safe to drink:

+ **Rainwater**: Rainwater can be obtained by placing a tarp, empty can, or any other type of clean, cup-shaped or concave container in a position to collect it. There are many naturally occurring options, such as firm leaves or a large rock with a depression.

+ **Plants with moisture inside**: Cacti, thistles, and birch trees are all examples of plants that can be cut open and squeezed or sucked to obtain drinking water. For maple trees, cut into the trunks and drain the sap.

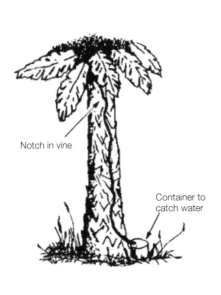

Notch in vine

Container to catch water

For vines, cut them as high as you can reach and drink the draining fluid.

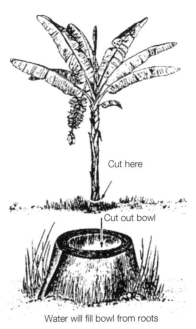

Cut here

Cut out bowl

Water will fill bowl from roots

For plantains, cut the trunk at the base and let water from its roots fill up the stump.

+ **Dew**: One method of obtaining water without having to decontaminate it is to collect dew. While it is always a good idea to decontaminate water obtained in nature, dew is generally a safe option. Tie rags or tufts of fine grass around your ankles and walk through dew-covered grass before sunrise. As the rags or grass tufts absorb the dew, wring the water into a container. Repeat the process until you have a supply of water or the dew is gone. Australian natives sometimes mop up as much as a liter an hour this way.

In a survival situation, you can even find water in other living things. Fish, for example, can provide you with many nutrients to keep you going, but also can provide fluid. There isn't a lot of fluid, but it may be just enough to keep your body and spirit going until you are rescued or locate another source of water. While the following steps may seem unappetizing, if you have no other options, this procedure may be able to keep you alive:

1. Hold the head and cut through the backbone near the tail.

2. Then tilt the head of the fish up, allowing the fluid to drain into your mouth or a collection receptacle.

3. You may also suck the fluid from the eyes of fish.

FOREST SHELTERS

There are many options when it comes to locating or building shelter in a forest, both natural and man-made. Differing seasons and weather should dictate where and how you address your need for shelter. As air cools it will dip into the low-lying areas and valleys, and warmer air will rise. So if you want to build your shelter to maximize natural heat, consider a place out of depressions and valleys, in the sunlight, and out of the wind. If you are seeking cooler temperatures, you can choose a lower-lying location as long as it isn't in an area with the potential for flooding. Use common sense and instinct when choosing a location, and try to remain in close proximity to water and fuel for fire.

Lean-to

A lean-to is built in heavily forested areas. It requires a limited amount of cordage to construct. The lean-to is an effective shelter, but does not offer a great degree of protection from the elements.

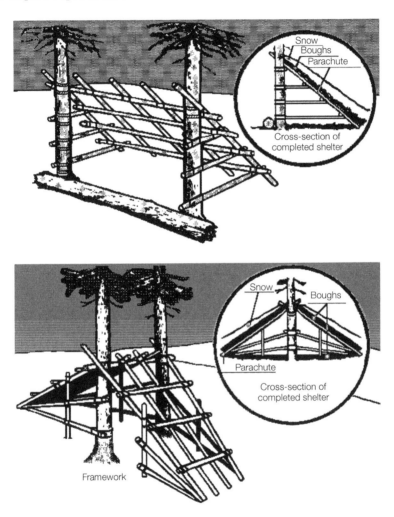

1. Select a site with two trees (4 to 12 inches in diameter), spaced far enough apart that a person can lay down between them. Two sturdy poles can be substituted by inserting them into the ground the proper distance apart.

2. Cut a pole to support the roof. It should be at least 3 to 4 inches in diameter and long enough to extend 4 to 6 inches past both trees. Tie the pole horizontally between the two trees, approximately 3 feet off the deck or ground.

3. Cut several long poles to be used as stringers. They are placed along the horizontal support bar approximately every 1½ feet and laid on the ground. All stringers may be tied to or laid on the horizontal support bar. A short wall of rocks or logs may be constructed on the ground to lift the stringers off the ground, creating additional height and inside space.

4. Cut several saplings and weave them horizontally between the stringers.

Sapling Shelter

A simple shelter that can be quickly built in an area where an abundance of saplings are growing is a sapling shelter, similar to the lean-to. This type of shelter is not practical in extreme heat or extreme cold, but in temperate weather is an excellent way to use the materials that are readily available to construct a safe place of refuge. To build a sapling shelter:

1. Find an area with two parallel rows of four to six saplings at least 4 feet long and approximately 1½ to 2 feet apart.

2. Clear the ground in between them.

3. Bend the saplings toward one another and lash their tops together, tying them to form several hoops. This will be the framework of the shelter.

4. Interweave additional branches between the saplings for added coverage and protection.

5. If you have a waterproof material (tarp, poncho, etc.) to lay over the top of the shelter, use it. If not, use leaves, brush, boughs, and snow to insulate and cover the shelter.

6. Close one end permanently. Hang material over the other end to form a door.

FOREST FOOD

The forest is full of edible plants and animals that can be used to not only survive, but also to provide sustenance for a long period of time. The key is knowing what to eat and what *not* to eat. That's not something that can be learned by trial and error. It's something that must be learned in advance or in reference material to avoid sickness or death. There are shelves in bookstores dedicated to real-life stories of survival where people were forced to rely on their surroundings to live. Sprinkled among them are the tragic tales of those who were ill-prepared and made poor decisions that led to tragic consequences. According to the *US Army Survival Manual*, "Nature can provide you with food that will let you survive any ordeal, if you don't eat the wrong plant. You must therefore learn as much as possible beforehand about the flora of the region where you will be operating."

The only way to determine if a plant is toxic is to use a field manual or the Universal Edibility Test (page 141). A few common misconceptions exist when it comes to identifying edible forest plants:

+ Eat what the animals eat. This is a dangerous guide, since many animals can eat things that are deadly to humans.

+ Boil plants to remove poison. While boiling a plant can remove certain toxins, it in no way guarantees that the plant is safe to consume.

+ Plants red in color are poisonous. This is a generalization that should not be used to determine a plant's toxicity. For example, poison oak, though red in fall and winter, is bright green in spring and summer, when it is just as toxic.

Edible Forest Animals

Most forest animals and insects can be eaten for some kind of nourishment. As with plants, though, it is best to be sure before consuming. Small animals are easily killed; you can harvest them by simply throwing a rock or stabbing them with a stick. Other animals, however, are harder to catch, and so are better suited to traps. There are some survival experts who question whether it is beneficial for a novice to attempt making a trap. Unless you know how to build one and what to use, and can be confident with its potential to catch game, it may not be worth the energy required.

Learn several ways to build simple snares and traps before any excursions into the woods. That knowledge can benefit you greatly when it comes time to locate food. Once you learn how to construct one, put that snare or trap near where the animal eats or drinks. Animals can be leery of a trap placed near their home. Your best options include:

+ **Young animals**: Most young animals are lean and flavorful, as with lamb and veal.

+ **Adult females**: Adult females tend to offer the most meat.

+ **Insects**: These are easily caught and surprisingly high in protein.

+ **Grubs**: Grubs are an easy source of protein, but avoid those found on the undersides of leaves

+ **Birds**: Birds are abundant and easily killed. If you can find a nest, eggs are a great source of protein.

+ **Fish**: Fish contain water as well as meat. Anywhere there is water, you're likely to find fish. Learn how to fashion a makeshift line and hook, or net.

MEDICINAL FOREST PLANTS

Lady fern: This fern is found all over North America, but thrives in wet, shaded areas. The leaves of the lady fern (and the related bracken fern) can be crushed into a mash in your hands and applied to skin to ease the pain of cuts and minor burns. The leaves can be cooked in a tea to treat cough, sore throat, and other throat or breathing afflictions.

Identification:

+ Fronds up to 20 inches long

+ Wedge shaped and lobed at apex

+ Brittle, shiny, delicate stalks

Catnip: This has been used for centuries to treat issues with the digestive system. The leaves are also crushed and worn as a natural insect repellent and applied directly to relieve itchy skin.

Identification:

- + 2 to 3 feet tall

- + Square, erect, branched stems

- + Heart-shaped and toothed leaves

- + Leaves are covered with fine, downy hairs, especially on the underside

- + Small, tubular two-lipped flowers

- + Flowers are white to lavender with reddish to purple spots

- + Minty fragrance

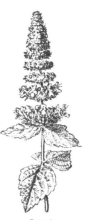

Catnip

Plantain: Plantain is extremely common and found in most parts of North America. The leaves are ground to treat irritated skin, such as bug bites, scrapes, and rashes. The chewed leaf can also be held in the mouth against a canker sore for pain relief.

Identification:

- + Grow to about 2 feet tall

- + Broad leaves that narrow at the stem

- + Three or five parallel veins diverge on the wide part of the leaf

- + Long, slender, densely flowered spikes growing from the middle of the plant

Jewelweed: This is also known as "touch me not" and is commonly used to treat poison ivy and other skin irritations such as eczema. The leaves are crushed and rubbed on the affected skin.

Identification:

- + 3 to 5 feet tall

- + Oval, toothed leaves

- + Trumpet-shaped flowers

+ Flowers are yellow or orange with red spots

+ Seeds will "pop" when touched (hence the name "touch me nots")

Burdock: Although not edible, the leaves of burdock are often used to treat burns and scalds. Chew or crush the leaves and blend with water and apply directly to mild burns. Also used on skin disorders such as diaper rash, cradle cap, and gout.

Identification:

+ 2 to 9 feet tall

+ Long, fleshy, gray-brown root (whitish on the inside)

+ Reddish pithy stem

+ Woolly branches

+ Heart-shaped leaves that are green and hairy on top, and downy gray on the bottom

+ Purple, thistle-like flowers across the top

+ Seedpods stick to clothing

CHAPTER 14
RESCUE OPERATIONS

Transporting a casualty is one of the most problematic aspects of combat casualty care. Military medics often require covering fire so they can move casualties in order to render care. Fortunately, in most situations you will not face enemy fire when rendering aid to someone, but some of the procedures used on the battlefield are useful for civilian situations as well.

One of the most difficult scenarios you may ever find yourself in is when you need to help remove another person from harm. It is often a dangerous situation, or the victim is in perilous terrain and cannot safely get themselves out of a bad spot. Having been a firefighter for almost 20 years, I have been in countless situations where I have been in a position to help a person or people when they are unable to get themselves to safety. I can tell you that, yes, anytime there is a catastrophic event, people will simply react and help out each other in the absence of emergency responders. But you should know that these scenarios lend themselves to additional injuries and casualties when untrained or unprepared people attempt a selfless act and end up becoming victims themselves. Whether or not you've had any formal training, you may find yourself in a situation where you will have to be the one to help. Learning and practicing rescue techniques will better prepare you for when the time comes and you need to make an instant decision to help someone.

The first thing that must be done in any type of rescue situation is a size-up (see page 10). You need to understand the situation as best you can before committing yourself to any type of aid. Be aware of the scope of the entire incident to best choose a course of action. Begin with the big picture. Has there been a catastrophic collapse of a structure, meaning there will be numerous victims that will need to be removed? Or has there been an isolated incident where someone experienced a medical emergency and they'll need to be moved to another location for treatment or transport? Each of those scenarios or anything in between will require you to make a quick assessment and then choose a course of action based on several things: your safety, the victim's safety, the mechanism of injury, extent of the injuries, and how best to move the person to safety.

YOUR SAFETY

You'll notice a common theme throughout this book is the safety of *you*, the rescuer. When it comes to rendering aid, your goal is to do the greatest good for the greatest number of people. That could mean just one person, but if you injure yourself helping them, you've essentially doubled the number of people who need help.

Be aware of your own physical fitness level. Lifting and moving people is no easy task. It's taxing on your muscles, and if not performed correctly could be harmful to your back. Self-awareness and a realistic knowledge of your own physical limitations can go a long way in preventing rescuer injury.

Evaluate the environment where the victim is located. Is the hazard that created the medical emergency still present? If not, is it safe for you to approach the person? Do you have medical gloves or leather gloves (depending on the situation)? Do you have eye protection, sturdy footwear, or any other personal protective equipment you may need for your specific circumstances? All of these things must be quickly assessed before your put yourself in a hazardous situation.

VICTIM SAFETY

Once you have deemed the scene safe for you to enter and offer assistance, do a quick evaluation on behalf of the victim similar to the one that you just did for yourself, without necessarily identifying their injuries yet. Are there any immediate hazards to the person? Hazards could be anything from a weakened structure or a downed power line to dangerous wildlife or even nearby broken glass that could cause further injury.

You should also identify paths of ingress and egress. Ensure there is a safe path of travel for you to get to the person and then to remove the person to where they can be further evaluated or treated. In the majority of medical situations, you're looking for things such as sharp corners or stairs that must be negotiated. In more severe instances, the hazards could be far greater, like fires and building collapse. Life safety is always the first priority in any circumstance. Once you have established rescuer and victim safety, you can begin a plan for moving the person or people to a safer location.

MECHANISM OF INJURY

Mechanism of injury (MOI) is another way of saying "what caused the person to be injured." Establishing the MOI will help to determine how best to move the victim. If it's a medical emergency, you can basically move them in any way that doesn't cause you harm and doesn't cause pain or further injury to the person. If the patient has sustained some form of trauma, there are further considerations that must be made due to the potential for a spinal injury.

If there is the chance for a neck or back injury to the patient, spinal precautions must be taken. Before you move them, their neck and back have to be stabilized, which takes further planning on your part. You'll need more time and more people to move someone with a suspected spinal injury. Determining what happened, the MOI, will dictate the method by which you move them.

EXTENT OF INJURIES

When you make contact with the patient you should determine the extent of their injuries before making any attempt to move them. The only exception would be a time-critical life-or-death situation—when immediate movement of the patient is necessary due to an imminent threat. In that case it is life over limb. Move the patient quickly to safety by whatever means is necessary.

When there isn't an immediate threat, identifying the patient's injuries will dictate the method by which you relocate them. Broken bones, for example, should be stabilized prior to moving the person. If they are unable to move themselves because of a medical condition such as a stroke or seizure, you have the freedom to use any type of carry that is most comfortable for them and easiest for you.

MOVING THE PATIENT

The goal of moving a sick or injured person should be to relocate them as safely as possible, for both the patient and rescuers, while making the patient as comfortable and secure as possible. If you have the option to recruit help in moving a person, you should do so. It reduces the risk of rescuer injury. You can, and should, assess what resources you have available. Take inventory of what you have available, such as people and items like chairs or blankets that can assist you.

The U.S. Air Force's *Self Aid and Buddy Care Instructor Handbook* states that before moving a victim, you must:

1. Check airway and respiration.

2. Evaluate type and extent of injury.

3. Ensure that bleeding is controlled and dressings are adequate.

4. Ensure bones are properly immobilized and supported.

In a best-case scenario, victims may be able to move themselves with little or no assistance. If the victim is not able to self-rescue, you'll have to evaluate the situation and determine the best and safest means to move them. The way you choose to remove a victim will depend on several factors:

+ How many victims are in need of rescue?

+ How many rescuers are available?

+ What is the size and condition of the victim(s)?

+ What are the conditions and capabilities of the rescuers?

+ What is the stability and safety of the immediate environment?

ONE-PERSON CARRIES

You may be the one and only available person who can help, or your group may have had to split up to assist multiple people. In either case, you find yourself acting alone and will want to choose the best method to move the patient to a safer area. One-person carries can be extremely punishing for the rescuer. There will be adrenaline working both for and against you. You may experience a surge of energy and strength, which lends itself to injury. You can easily pull a back muscle or sprain your ankle. It's also common, after a rush of adrenaline, to suddenly "run out of gas." All of your energy is spent quickly, and then you begin to fatigue and experience a rapid decrease in strength. Often rescuers will compensate by relying on tired larger muscle groups, like back muscles, to perform the brunt of the work, which exposes the rescuer to injury. You should utilize multiple rescuers when possible. Which carry you choose depends on the patient's comfort and the ability of the rescuer or rescuers. The U.S. Air Force's *Self Aid and Buddy Care Instructor Handbook* identifies the best ways to move a victim:

One-person walk assist: If the victim simply needs help walking out, begin by helping them to their feet. Have the victim place his or her arm around your neck and hold on to their wrist. Place your other hand around their waist and assist them out of the dangerous area, moving as cautiously as the situation allows so as not to cause greater injury.

Cradle-in-arms carry: If the victim is a child or a small adult, you may be able to perform a cradle-in-arms carry. Kneel beside the child and place one arm around their back and one under their thighs. Lift slightly and roll the child into the hollow formed by your arms and chest. Lift with your leg muscles and carefully stand.

Arm carry: Reach around the victim's back and under their knees. They may be able to assist by putting an arm around your neck. Lift carefully with your legs and not your back. Despite how easy this looks in the movies, it should only be performed if the rescuer is very strong and the victim is not too large.

Firefighter carry: This method is used to carry someone over long distances. This is another carry that should only be done by a very strong rescuer with a smaller victim. It is difficult to move a victim who is on the ground into the proper position to be carried. With the victim in the lying position, hook your elbows under their armpits and raise them to a standing position. Place your right leg between the victim's legs. Grab their right hand with your left. Squat down and wrap your right arm around the victim's right knee. Rise up and raise the victim's right thigh over your right shoulder. Carry them to safety.

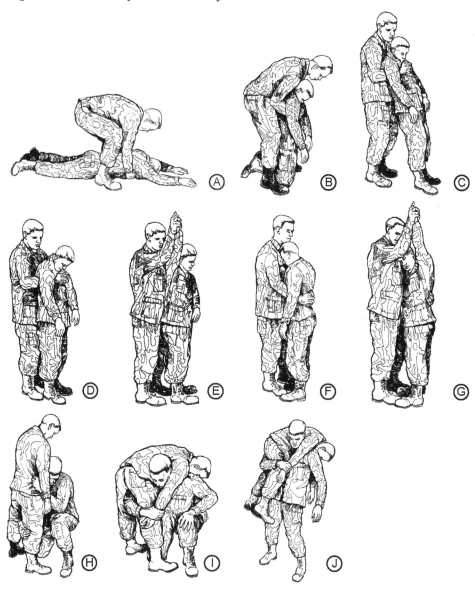

Firefighter carry starting with victim lying on stomach

Pack-strap carry: This carry could potentially be uncomfortable for the victim. Place the victim's arms over your shoulders. Cross the victim's arms, grasping the opposite wrists, and pull them close to your chest. Squat slightly and drive your hips into the victim while bending at the waist. Balance the load on your hips as you lift up and carry.

Saddleback carry: The victim must be conscious to perform this carry because they must be able to hold the rescuer. Raise the victim to an upright position. Place an arm around the victim's waist and move to their side. Have the victim place an arm around your neck as you move in front of them. Have the victim then encircle their other arm around your neck. Stoop and raise the victim up onto your back, lifting with your legs. Clasp your hands under their thighs and carry them to safety.

TWO-PERSON CARRIES

Two-person walk assist: Each rescuer stands on either side of the victim and helps them to the standing position. Once they are fully upright, drape the victim's arms across the rescuers' shoulders. Each rescuer puts their inside arm around the victim's back and links it to the other rescuer's arm. Assist the victim in walking to safety at their speed.

Chair carry: If you have a sturdy chair available, this method makes moving the victim much easier. Place the victim in a chair. The rescuer at the head grabs the chair, palms in from the back, and then leans the chair back on its hind legs. The second rescuer grabs the front legs of the chair. For short distances or on stairs, the second rescuer should face in. Over longer distances, he or she should face out. At the command of the person at the head, stand and carry the victim out.

Two-person extremity carry (fore-and-aft carry): Help the victim to a seated position. The first rescuer kneels behind the victim and reaches under their arms, assuming the bulk of the victim's weight. The rescuer's forearms should be at the armpits of the victim, and they should secure their hold by grasping the victim's wrists. (This rescuer can grasp their own wrists, but holding the wrists of the victim helps reduce the likelihood that the victim will slip through the arms of the rescuer.) The second rescuer backs in between the victim's legs and grabs behind the knees. At the command of the rescuer at the head, stand using your legs, and remove the victim.

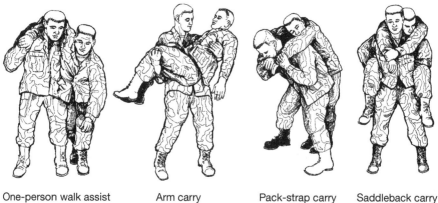

One-person walk assist   Arm carry   Pack-strap carry   Saddleback carry

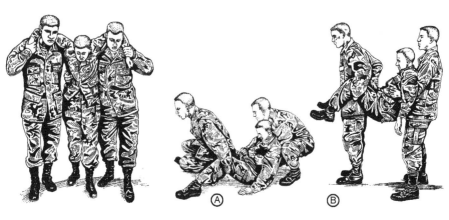

Two-person walk assist   Two-person extremity carry

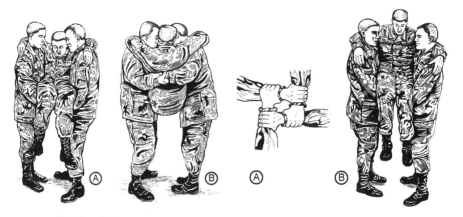

Two-handed seat carry   Four-handed seat carry

Two-handed seat carry: The two- and four-handed carries should only be performed on fully conscious victims. To perform the two-handed seat carry, each rescuer kneels on either side of the victim. Raise the victim to the seated position and link arms behind their back. Place your free arms under the victim's knees and link arms. As you stand together, have the victim place their arms around the rescuers for support.

Four-handed seat carry: Each rescuer will grab their own right wrist with their left hand. The two rescuers then grasp the left forearm of the other rescuer with their right hand. The rescuers squat down and allow the fully conscious victim to sit down on their interlocked hands. It is helpful if the victim can wrap their arms around the rescuers to assist with stability and balance. The rescuers then carefully stand and walk to safety.

LITTER CARRY

Often there will be items or even debris around that you can use to your advantage. If you can locate two "poles" and a blanket, curtain, or any other piece of fabric large enough, you can quickly build an improvised stretcher to carry victims who aren't ambulatory. There are multiple ways to construct a makeshift stretcher. Utilizing an improvised stretcher will require a minimum of two rescuers, and could use as many as six. Your first task is to locate the "poles." They can be sturdy pieces of lumber, tent poles, curtain rods, roof rack supports, or any other items that are sturdy enough to support the weight of a victim. Next you must find the fabric that makes up the middle part of the stretcher. You'll want to find a blanket, tarp, sleeping bag, or any other fabric that can be used to support body weight.

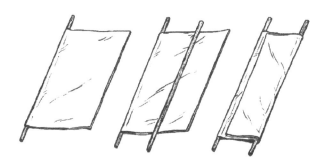

1. Lay the blanket or other material flat on the ground.

2. Lay your "poles" about one foot on either side of the center of the blanket.

3. Ensure there is enough pole sticking out of either end for the rescuers to comfortably hold.

4. Fold one side of the cloth so that it reaches the other side.

5. Fold the other side back over the poles.

6. Continue to fold the fabric around the spaced poles as needed.

A second method is to:

1. Fold the large piece of fabric in half.

2. Place the first pole in the middle of the fabric.

3. Fold the fabric in half again so that the pole is in the fold.

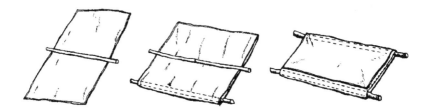

4. Place the second pole in the middle of the fabric parallel to the first.

5. Fold the fabric over the second pole back toward the first.

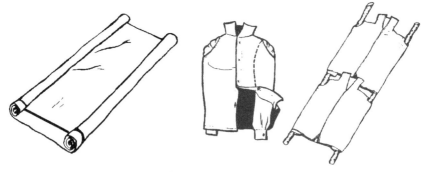

Other improvised litters

To transfer a victim to a litter, you should follow these steps:

1. The four bearers take their positions. Bearer number 2 stands at the victim's ankle, bearer number 3 stands at the victim's shoulder, and bearers number 4 and 1 stand on either side of the victim's hips.

2. Each bearer kneels on the knee that is nearest the casualty's feet. Bearer number 2 put his forearms under the legs, bearers 1 and 4 put their arms under the small of the back, and bearer number 3 puts one hand under the neck and to the farther armpit and the other hand under the nearer shoulder. All bearers lift the patient slowly and carefully and place him on the knees of bearers number 2, 3, and 4.

3. As soon as the patient is firmly supported on the knees of bearers number 2, 3, and 4, bearer number 1 reaches for the litter and slides it beneath the casualty, against the ankles of the other bearers. Bearer number 1 then holds the litter in place as bearers 2, 3, and 4 lower the victim gently onto the litter.

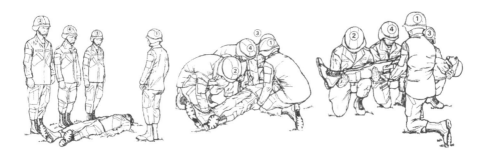

If there are only two bearers available, you should follow these steps to transfer a victim to a litter:

1. Begin with the litter already open and on the ground near the patient. Bearers number 1 and 2 take their positions. Bearer number 1 stands at the patient's thigh, and bearer number 2 stands at the shoulder.

2. Each barer kneels on the knee that is nearest the casualty's feet. Bearer number 1 puts his arms under the hips and knees, while bearer number 2 puts his arms under the back.

3. Both bearers lift the patient slowly and carefully and place him on their knees. They readjust their hold, rise to their feet, and move as close as possible to the side of the litter.

4. Both bearers kneel and again place the casualty on their knees. They then gently lower the patient onto the litter.

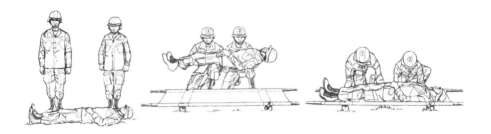

If the casualty is conscious and able, there is another way of loading a patient onto a litter. Bearers number 1 and 2 stand on either side of the casualty's hips. They then kneel on the knee nearest to the patient's feet, grasp each other's left forearms under the victim's knees, and grasp each other's right forearms under the victim's armpits and behind the back. The casualty puts their arms around the necks of the bearers. The bearers move the patient above a litter, with each bearer standing on either side. They kneel again, lowering the patient onto the litter in a sitting position. The patient releases hold of the bearers' necks once sitting safely on the litter. Both bearers assist the patient in lying down.

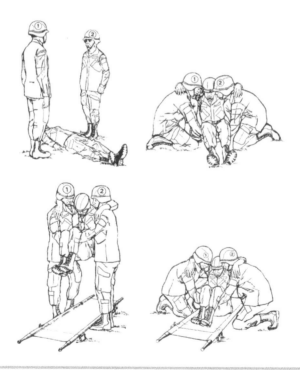

Lifting the Litter

Depending on the specific injury and how many rescuers are available, there are different ways to lift the litter and move the victim. If there is a suspected spinal injury and more than two rescuers, at least one rescuer should hold the victim's head to prevent movement that could potentially cause further damage.

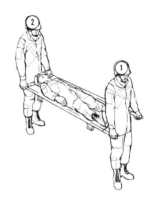

Two rescuers: One rescuer goes to the head of the litter and the other to the foot. They then lift together on the 1, 2, 3 count of the rescuer at the head.

Three rescuers: This is the same as the two-rescuer lift, but the third rescuer should hold the victim's head.

Four rescuers: Two rescuers stand on either side of the victim. (If a spinal injury is suspected, one rescuer should hold the victim's head, while two rescuers carry the head of the litter and one carries the foot.)

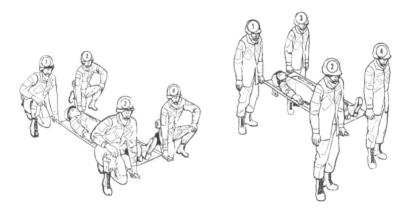

If a fractured spine is suspected, bearer number 1 should keep the patient's head straight and still rather than supporting the patient's weight or opening the litter. Bearer number 3 should reach underneath the casualty and pull the litter towards the bearers with one hand.

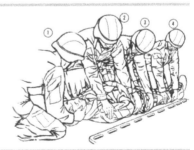

DRAGS

There are scenarios where assisting or carrying someone to safety is simply not possible. Time, terrain, or a lack of people available to assist can hinder any notions of a methodical removal. In such cases, you must quickly "grab 'n' go." Dragging a victim is a last resort. The environment is usually treacherous, making everything dangerous for both the victim and the rescuer. The safer option is to conduct a coordinated carry from a dangerous area to a secure location. However, when the situation dictates you drag a victim to safety, there are a few ways to do it:

Shoulder drag: Place the victim in the seated position and align yourself behind. Squat down and reach under the victim's arms. Grab their right wrist with your left hand and their left wrist with your right. From the squatted position, stand, pulling the victim's back into your chest. Rise up with your legs rather than your back, and drag the victim to safety.

Cradle drop drag: This is effective in moving a victim up or down steps. 1) Kneel at the victim's head (with him lying on his back). 2) Slide your hands, with palms up, under the victim's shoulders and get a firm hold under his armpits. 3) Rise (partially), supporting the victim's head on one of your forearms. (You may bring your elbows together and let the victim's head rest on both of your forearms.) Rise and drag the victim backward. (The victim is in a semisitting position.) 4) Back down the steps, supporting the victim's head and body and letting his hips and legs drop from step to step. If the victim needs to be moved up the steps, you should back up the steps using the same procedure.

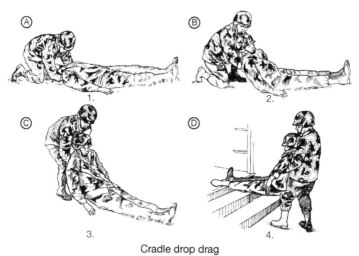

Cradle drop drag

Blanket drag: Locate a blanket, curtain, tarp, or any other large piece of fabric. Tuck the blanket under the victim and roll the victim on to the center. Grasp the blanket behind the victim's head and drag them clear of the hazard.

Feet drag: Dragging a victim by their feet is basically the last resort of the last resorts. Use it when you have no other way to move the victim, but need to get them to a safer place. Place the victim on their back. Squat and grab the victim by the ankles, stand, and pull. Ideally you'll pull them across a smooth, flat surface, but rarely in a disaster situation will you find one. Understand that when you drag a victim in this manner, their head is prone to injury, and their arms will drag away from their body, likely catching on doorways and debris. Do your best to limit the additional injuries to the victim as you remove them from harm.

Neck drag: This particular drag will allow you to drag a victim while keeping a low profile. It is often used by soldiers behind concealment. Tie the victim's hands together at the wrists.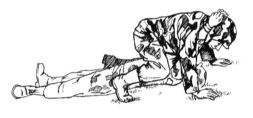 Straddle the victim in a kneeling face-to-face position. Loop the victim's tied hands over and around your neck. Crawl forward, dragging the victim with you.

Note: Do not drag a victim by the wrists. It will cause joint separation, among other problems. The weight of a human body is too great for the wrist.

CHAPTER 15

PSYCHOLOGICAL FIRST AID

Medical first aid has been a topic of discussion, evaluation, and education for as long as humans have been injuring themselves and each other. Perhaps the first caveman to drop a rock on his foot grunted for assistance. The other cave people, through trial and error, determined what the best actions were to aid someone who had dropped a rock on their foot. Since then we have studied, improved, studied some more, and improved some more in all areas of medicine. Just think how far humans have come in the field of medical treatment in the last century alone. A hundred years ago, common yet ineffective methods of treating battle injuries led to countless wounded soldiers needlessly losing their lives, yet progress was being made. The early 1900s gave us the first splints used for broken bones, the introduction of medical sanitation, the advent of the rudimentary X-ray, and the treatment of patients according to the severity of their injury rather than their rank.

Around 1914 another medical issue began to arise. Soldiers coined the term "shell shock." Army doctors were struggling to understand what was happening to soldiers who showed no visible signs of medical injury, yet displayed symptoms such as tremors, fatigue, confusion, and nightmares. When soldiers showed the physical symptoms and were unable to function, yet no obvious cause could be identified, they were labeled as suffering from shell shock. At that time, anyone showing signs of shell shock was considered a coward. The condition's symptoms were very similar to the modern diagnosis of post-traumatic stress disorder (PTSD).

Unfortunately, is wasn't until the last few decades that serious study of the effects of traumatic events and mental treatment really began to take shape. The term "post-traumatic stress disorder" was coined in the early 1970s to describe the symptoms of returning veterans of the Vietnam War, but wasn't officially recognized by the American Psychiatric Association until 1980. "Shell shock," "combat fatigue," and "war neurosis" are all trauma-related mental disorders that fall under the current definition of PTSD.

It was during studies in the '70s and '80s that doctors began to recognize the effects of a single traumatic event or the culmination of many. They studied the causes, effects, and treatments, and that research continues today to better understand and treat PTSD.

PTSD is most often associated with members of the military, where the studies began due to the immense trauma soldiers had experienced and continue to experience. Lately, however, experts are understanding that PTSD can affect anyone. How you process and respond to a traumatic event is not a measure of mental toughness or how "strong" of a person you are. It's the result of many combined factors like age, physical health, previous experience, and emotional stability at the time. Traumatic events occur every day. Anything from the unexpected death of a family member or friend to a car accident can lead to mental side effects that can have long-term consequences.

Men and women in the military, along with emergency responders, doctors, nurses, and a variety of other professions, find themselves dealing with trauma and death on an almost daily basis. That does not mean, however, that they will necessarily suffer from PTSD, just as it does not mean that you *won't* suffer from PTSD after some isolated incident. The most important thing is to acknowledge that it's a very real and corrosive disorder that can hit a person suddenly without warning, or it can be a slow, insidious process that manifests itself over time.

The U.S. military *Leaders' Manual for Combat Stress Control* warns, "Future combat will strain human endurance to unprecedented levels. If these challenges are left unchecked by poor mental and physical conditioning of soldiers, they could result in the disastrous failure of entire units." This also can be said of civilians placed in traumatic situations such as natural disasters.

STRESS

Believe it or not, we need stress because it has many positive benefits. Stress provides us with challenges; it gives us chances to learn about our values and strengths. Stress can show our ability to handle pressure without breaking; it tests our adaptability and flexibility; and it can stimulate us to do our best. Some people say they thrive under pressure, that the stress they feel when up against a deadline or other pressure causes them to simply react rather than overthink.

Because we usually don't consider unimportant events stressful, stress can also be an excellent indicator of the significance we attach to an event. In other words, it highlights what's important to us. We actually need to have some stress in our lives, but too much of anything can be bad. The goal is to have a healthy amount of stress, but not an excess of it. Too much stress can take its toll on a person or organization. Too much stress leads to distress. Distress causes an uncomfortable tension that we try to escape and, preferably, avoid.

Signs and Symptoms

The following are a few of the common signs of distress you may find in someone else or yourself when faced with too much stress:

+ Difficulty making decisions

+ Angry outbursts

+ Forgetfulness

+ Low energy level

+ Constant worrying

+ Propensity for mistakes

+ Thoughts about death or suicide

+ Trouble getting along with others

+ Withdrawing from others

+ Hiding from responsibilities

+ Carelessness

Traumatic stress may affect a person's cognitive functioning, meaning decision-making becomes difficult. A person can quickly become overwhelmed and not be able to make a decision, or they may feel complete apathy toward something that should be important to them. They may act out irrationally in ways that are out of character, becoming easily agitated or, again, apathetic. Curious memory gaps develop concerning day-to-day events, a condition known as dissociative amnesia. Basic behaviors can be altered to the point where others might say, "They're just not themselves."

Physical health can be affected as well. Blood flow to the brain surges under traumatic stress and can lead to sustained high blood pressure. Often as a coping mechanism or as a form of emotional escape, someone experiencing traumatic stress may turn to alcohol or drug use. An overuse quickly leads to dependency. Depression and lethargy create a propensity for obesity and tobacco use. Energy levels are often decreased following a traumatic event. There are also multiple medical conditions that are tied to post-traumatic stress such as dementia, chronic pain, autoimmune disease, irritable bowel syndrome, and liver disease. Physical health and mental health are closely related, and caring for one should not mean neglecting the other.

The *US Army Survival Manual* addresses stress, stating it can be constructive or destructive. Stress can inspire you to operate successfully and perform at your maximum efficiency, but it can also cause you to panic and forget all your experience and training. The key to coping is your ability to manage the inevitable stresses you'll encounter. The survivor is the person who works with his stresses instead of letting his stresses work on him.

RECOGNIZING PTSD

Humans have been able to survive many shifts in our environment throughout the centuries. Our ability to adapt physically and mentally to a changing world kept us alive while other species around us gradually died off. However, these survival mechanisms that can help us can also work against us if we don't understand and anticipate their presence. It's not surprising that the average person will have some psychological reactions in a traumatic situation.

Even the *US Army Survival Manual* discusses traumatic stress as part of its survival training and encourages military personnel to be able to recognize it in themselves and each other. The same awareness must be practiced by you and those around you, particularly if one or all of you have sustained a traumatic incident. All too often we either suppress the feelings that come along with post-traumatic stress, telling ourselves to "get over it," or we succumb to them and are overwhelmed with a feeling of hopelessness. Either reaction can be just as dangerous as the other. PTSD can lead to addiction, depression, self-harm, harming others, or a variety of other dangerous responses.

Post-traumatic stress can manifest itself in a variety of ways. It can be felt in both physical and psychological symptoms. The physical symptoms can sometimes be wrongly attributed to a medical condition, but thanks to modern studies, these, along with recognizable psychological symptoms, today often lead to proper PTSD diagnosis and treatment.

Signs and Symptoms

As a firefighter I am keenly aware of the symptoms of post-traumatic stress. I've seen them in my friends and coworkers, and experienced them myself. Thanks to proper training and recognition, my fire department and most other organizations take a proactive approach to treating post-traumatic stress. We learn the symptoms to watch for and the steps to take in response. Following are some symptoms that you may experience yourself or take note of a friend or loved one experiencing. Remember, the person feeling the effects of post-traumatic stress does not have to feel all of these things. In fact, it could be a single symptom listed below, or simply the acknowledgment that something is bothersome that should warrant action to begin treatment as early as possible.

Physical symptoms of trauma:

+ Fatigue

+ Increased alcohol or drug consumption

+ Sleep disturbances

+ Headache

+ Loss of appetite

+ Hyperactivity

+ Nightmares

+ Diarrhea

+ Stomach pain or nausea

+ Chest pain

+ Psychological symptoms of trauma

+ Sadness or depression

+ Relationship strife

+ Mood swings

+ Feelings of helplessness

+ Fear of reoccurrence

+ Irritability

+ Isolation or withdrawal

+ Inability to concentrate

+ Self-blame

+ Feeling numb

Any event can lead to stress and, as everyone has experienced, events don't always come one at a time. Often, stressful events occur simultaneously. These events are not stress, but they produce it and are called "stressors." Stressors are the obvious cause, while stress is the response. Once the body recognizes the presence of a stressor, it begins to act to protect itself. In response to a stressor, the body prepares either to "fight or flee," which involves an internal SOS sent throughout the body. As the body responds to this SOS, several actions take place. The body releases stored fuels (sugar and fats) to provide quick energy; breathing rate increases to supply more oxygen to the blood; muscle tension increases to prepare for action; blood clotting mechanisms are activated to reduce bleeding from cuts; senses become more acute (hearing becomes more sensitive, eyes become big, smell becomes sharper) so that you're more aware of your surroundings; and heart rate and blood pressure rise to provide more blood to the muscles.

This protective posture lets a person cope with potential dangers; however, a person cannot maintain such a level of alertness indefinitely. Stressors are not courteous; one stressor does not leave because another one arrives. Stressors add up. The cumulative effect of minor stressors can become a major distress if they all happen too close together. As the body's resistance to stress wears down and the sources of stress continue or increase, eventually a state of exhaustion arrives. At this point, the ability to resist stress or use it in a positive way gives out, and signs of distress appear. Anticipating stressors and developing strategies to cope with them are two ingredients in the effective management of stress.

Treatment

Just because someone encounters a traumatic event does not mean that they will suffer PTSD. There are normal responses to trauma. Nightmares, depressing thoughts, and feelings of fear are all expected responses that can fade over time. It's when they don't or when symptoms worsen that someone must intervene. Psychological aid must be given appropriately just as first aid is.

Treating post-traumatic stress disorder is going to vary from person to person. Treatments can range from a simple counseling session to long-term psychological care and possibly medication. Caring for PTSD means not fighting the symptoms, but working with the feelings. The symptoms are an indication of an underlying issue. There has been a psychological trauma that, despite what many believe, don't just "go away." The trauma has the potential to lie festering beneath the surface for any length of time and can reveal itself in sometimes tragic ways. Encourage those who have experienced a traumatic event to express their feelings to help avoid "emotional overload." There are both mental and physical benefits from engaging in open and honest conversation. The U.S. military is being both proactive and reactive by addressing soldier stress in both preparation and training, as well as post-operational periods.

To help someone who has experienced traumatic stress you should: Brief the person or people on what to expect to see and feel as they conduct their operations; emphasize teamwork to ease the workload and diffuse emotional overload; rotate personnel; ensure proper hydration and nutrition; and encourage breaks. These steps won't eliminate all the effects of PTSD, but may mitigate some of the long-term effects before they begin.

In Ernest Hemingway's famous book *For Whom the Bell Tolls*, a woman, Maria, is troubled by a brutally traumatic event that happened to her earlier in life. She has recently married a man and is not sure if or how to tell her new husband about it. Maria receives advice from another woman about how to handle the situation, and then explains to her husband, "She said I could tell thee of what was done to me if I ever began to think of it again because thou art a good man and have already understood it all. But that it were better to never speak of it unless it came back to me as a black thing as it had been before and then that telling of thee might rid me of it." What she's saying is that it isn't necessary to go back and relive the memory and deal with it, but if that memory continues to come back as that "black thing," it may be beneficial to talk to a trusted person about it. That trusted person could be a friend or family member, but if that "black thing" continues, professional counseling should be sought out.

Mental-health professionals use techniques such as:

+ **Cognitive therapy**: identifies dysfunctional thinking and emotional responses and works to modify them

+ **Exposure therapy**: exposes the person to the traumatic issue in a safe environment while the professional works to reduce anxiety

+ **Anxiety management**: could be a wide range of treatments, from general counseling to medication

Psychological first aid is every bit as important as medical aid and all too often gets overlooked. The best way to treat a mental issue is to identify it and seek help. Be aware of the symptoms, both in yourself and in others. If you or someone you know has experienced a traumatic event, pay attention to the subtleties in behavior. Do you or they mention trouble sleeping or eating? Is there a change in behavior? Do you or they seem uncharacteristically distracted or removed? Once you have identified that there may be an issue, the absolute best thing that can be done is to get professional help. It is not a sign of weakness. I know of many cases where my coworkers reluctantly sought help and were extremely grateful they did, and I also know cases where they didn't get help and there were long-term consequences. Know the symptoms and get the help so that the healing process can happen.

If you're in a crisis situation, professional psychological aid is likely not going to be available until well after the incident has de-escalated. Also keep in mind that just because someone isn't showing debilitating signs of traumatic stress, that doesn't mean they aren't affected. Everyone who has been touched by the event has been affected in one way or another. There are things you can do to relieve stress until professional care can be obtained.

+ Limit the post-disaster work being done by those directly affected.

+ Encourage peer partners and peer consultation.

+ Ensure enough rest, nutrition, and hydration.

+ Use stress management tools such as relaxation techniques and identifying when someone is HALT (hungry, angry, lonely, or tired).

+ Practice religious faith, philosophy, or spirituality.

+ Continue to reassure, console, and monitor for changes as needed.

CHAPTER 16

RESUSCITATION

Can there be a more critical and stressful situation than when you're faced with someone you love who has stopped breathing and whose heart has stopped beating? According to the American Heart Association (AHA), there are over 326,000 out-of-hospital incidents of cardiac arrest annually in the United States. Of those, 90 percent are fatal. It's a sad and sobering fact. Cardiac arrest is basically when something disrupts the blood flow to the brain, lungs, and other organs—a leading cause of death in adults. The odds are not good for someone who experiences cardiac arrest outside of a hospital setting, and it is in the critical moments when someone becomes unresponsive that a bystander's response could mean the difference between life and death.

AIRWAY POSITIONING

When you're checking to see if an unconscious person is breathing and find that they are not, a simple airway reposition could possibly allow spontaneous respirations. Check for a pulse at the wrist or neck.

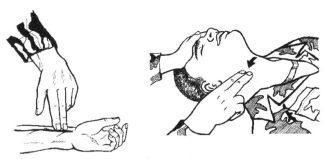

How to check for a pulse

Look for chest rise, and put your face down near the face of the patient, and feel for exhalations.

If you don't feel any, and don't see their chest rise, perform what is called a head tilt/chin lift. As long as there has been no trauma, this maneuver could allow breathing to return.

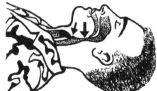

Checking for breathing

Head Tilt/Chin Lift

1. Position yourself beside the patient's head.

2. Place one hand firmly on the patient's forehead and apply pressure so that their head tilts back.

3. Place the fingers of your other hand on the bony part of the chin.

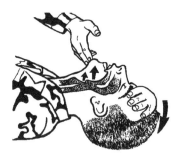

4. Lift the chin upward while keeping your other hand on the forehead, maintaining the tilt.

If there is obvious or suspected trauma, you should avoid moving the cervical spine. The head tilt/chin lift should be abandoned in favor of the jaw-thrust maneuver, which allows you to reposition the airway without compromising the neck.

Head tilt/chin lift

Jaw-Thrust Maneuver

1. Position yourself at the patient's head.

2. Place your fingers behind the angle of the jaw and lift the jaw upward.

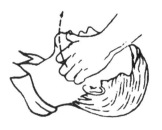

3. Use your thumbs to open the patient's mouth to allow breathing through the mouth as well as the nose.

Jaw-thrust maneuver

CHAIN OF SURVIVAL

Immediate CPR can double or triple someone's chance of survival. According to the AHA, there are sequential steps that need to occur in a timely manner to give someone the best possible odds of survival when they suffer out-of-hospital cardiac arrest. These steps are called the "Chain of Survival." When cardiac arrest occurs, the situation is grave. The patient's heart has stopped beating and death is imminent. Steps *must* be taken in order to give the person any chance of survival. The Chain of Survival consists of:

1. Early recognition

2. High-quality CPR

3. Rapid defibrillation

4. Rapid transport

5. Advanced cardiac care

Early Recognition

Early recognition is vitally important. Without oxygenated blood, tissue begins to die almost immediately and death occurs quickly. When someone suffers cardiac arrest, the best possible outcomes will begin when someone recognizes it and takes action. The absolute first thing that should be done is to call 911 and retrieve a defibrillator if there is one available. Rather than shout out "Someone call 911!," designate a specific person to make the call, and yet another person (if there are other bystanders willing to assist) to retrieve a defibrillator while you begin the next steps.

SIGNS AND SYMPTOMS OF CARDIAC ARREST

+ Chest pain

+ Light-headedness/dizziness

+ Nausea

+ Shortness of breath

+ Other pain such as in the jaw or arm

Women tend to experience additional "non-typical" symptoms of cardiac arrest, such as pressure in the upper back, malaise (fatigue), and fainting.

High-Quality CPR

The 2015 AHA guidelines recommend that if a bystander is not CPR-certified, they can best help by performing "hands-only CPR." Most people feel helpless during a cardiac emergency. They are cautious or even afraid to act because they don't know CPR, are afraid they may hurt the victim, or are simply overwhelmed by the gravity of the situation. By approving and recommending hands-only CPR, the AHA has effectively reduced the stress level of responders who, without "mouth to mouth," are more likely to administer *high-quality CPR*, thus increasing the survival rate of victims.

When someone experiences cardiac arrest, they will typically become unresponsive and collapse. You should approach them and "shake and shout." Shake their arm and ask if they are OK. If you get no response, immediately initiate chest compressions. Sometimes someone asks, "What if they don't need CPR?" If they show no visible signs of movement or breathing, err on the side of administering CPR. Studies have shown that it is highly unlikely that you could cause long-term harm, and if their heart is not beating, the immediate, high-quality chest compressions could be exactly what saves their life.

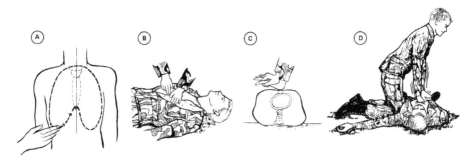

Hand placement for chest thrust: locating the xiphoid process
(A, B) and hand position on chest (C, D)

To perform chest thrusts, place the unresponsive patient on his back, face up, and open his mouth. Kneel close to the side of the patient's body. Place the palm of one hand firmly on the victim's sternum, the flat area between the breasts where the ribs come together. Located at the bottom is a small, bony notch called the xiphoid process. Try to place your hand slightly (approximately the width of two fingers) above the xiphoid process.

Place your other hand on top of the first and interlace your fingers. You fingers should be slightly raised so that the primary contact being made is between your palm and the victim's sternum. At that point, the AHA recommends to push hard and fast. Ideally, for an adult, you will want to push about 2 inches into the chest. Will you break ribs? Probably. It is common for ribs to break or to become separated from the sternum, but this is a small price to pay if the end result is a life saved. It can be difficult, depending on the person, to compress the full 2 inches. Using your body weight will help you push deeper and not fatigue as quickly. Align your torso directly above your hands and compress straight down.

Currently, experts teach that you should compress the chest to the rate of the hit disco song "Staying Alive," which has roughly the same number of beats per minute that is recommended for adult CPR. Studies have shown that people feel more confident when they are able to remember the rate by compressing to the beat of a familiar song.

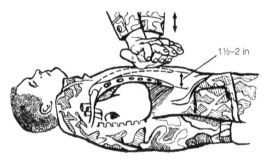

Chest compressions   Rescue breaths

Even though the American Heart Association stresses calling 911 and immediately beginning compressions only, if you are trained to do so you can administer rescue breaths as well. After giving 30 chest compressions, give two breaths, each lasting one second. Pinch the victim's nose and blow into their mouth strongly enough for you to see the victim's chest rise. Stop every two minutes (four cycles of 30:2) to check for a pulse. If there is no pulse, continue CPR.

Children and infants: When CPR is needed on an adult, it is a stressful situation for any rescuer involved, but when the victim is a child (one to eight years old) or infant (less than one year old), the stress seems to escalate astronomically. The CPR process for children and infants is similar to that for adults, but it does vary slightly. As long as you are trained to do so, administer a compression to breaths ratio of 30:2, the same as that for adults. The difference lies in the compressions. When giving compressions to a child, align your hand the same way you would with an adult, but compress with only one hand rather than two, and compress one-third the depth of the chest. For an infant, put your index finger across the nipple line and then, using your middle and ring finger, compress one-third the depth of the infant's chest. Always compress at a rate of about 100 beats per minute.

Rapid Defibrillation

A major element of returning a pulse to someone who has experienced cardiac arrest is *rapid defibrillation*. Most schools, churches, businesses, and offices have an Automated External Defibrillator (AED) on the premises. When you recognize someone in need of CPR, send someone to retrieve the nearest AED. Although it is recommended that you obtain proper training, even if you haven't attended a class on the operation of an AED, they have been made to be extremely simple to operate, with built-in safety features. When immediate CPR begins, for every minute between collapse and defibrillation, the survival rate decreases 3 to 4 percent (without immediate CPR, that number falls 7 to 10 percent per minute).

The AED contains two patches that are large oval stickers. On each sticker will be a picture of where exactly to place it on the body of the victim. Turn the AED on and then the voice prompts will walk you through the rest of the process. To ease any fears, know that it will not allow you to shock someone who does not need it.

Rapid Transport and Advanced Cardiac Care

The arriving ambulance will provide *rapid transport* and take the patient to a hospital where they will receive the *advanced cardiac care* they require. Unfortunately, only 39 percent of the people who experience out-of-hospital cardiac arrest will receive the immediate care they need. By starting the Chain of Survival as quickly as possible, you will help the victim receive the best possible odds to survive a dire situation.

Qualified CPR and AED classes are the best way to learn the latest AHA-recommended guidelines, practice performing CPR, and gain confidence to know that you are certified to perform the necessary steps that may save a life.

A difficult reality to acknowledge is that when someone's heart stops beating and they stop breathing, despite what the movies would have you believe, survival is a statistical long shot. When one person suffers cardiac arrest, you and those around you can rally around them and provide immediate care. During a disaster, however, when there are numerous casualties, CPR is not an option. Unfortunately, CPR is time-consuming and labor-intensive, and is not performed in a mass-casualty incident unless there are enough rescuers to do it without neglecting other viable patients. Remember, your goal is to do the greatest amount of good for the greatest number of people, and when there are more injured people than there are personnel to take care of them, the ones who have no heartbeat are to be considered deceased.

REFERENCES

FIELD MANUALS

Bureau of Medicine and Surgery. *Manual of Naval Preventive Medicine: Prevention of Heat and Cold Stress Injuries.* NAVMED P-5010-3, Rev. 2-2009. Washington, D.C.: U.S. Government Printing Office, 2009.

Department of the Air Force. *Infection Prevention and Control Program.* By Dorothy A. Hogg. AFI44-108. Washington, D.C.: U.S. Government Printing Office, 2015.

Department of the Air Force. *Self Aid and Buddy Care Instructor Handbook.* By D. B. Bayliss and L. J. Stierle. AFH 36-2218, Vol 1. Washington, D.C.: U.S. Government Printing Office, 1996.

Department of the Army. *The Aidman's Medical Guide.* FM 8-36. Washington, D.C.: U.S. Government Printing Office, 1973.

Department of the Army. *Altitude Acclimatization and Illness Management.* TB MED 505. Washington, D.C.: U.S. Government Printing Office, 2010.

Department of the Army. *Casualty Evacuation.* ATP 4-25.13. Washington, D.C.: U.S. Government Printing Office, 2013.

Department of the Army. *Control of Hazards to Health from Laser Radiation.* TB MED 524. Washington, D.C.: U.S. Government Printing Office, 2006.

Department of the Army. *Foot Marches.* FM 21-18. Washington, D.C.: U.S. Government Printing Office, 1990.

Department of the Army. *Jungle Operations*. FM 90-5. Washington, D.C.: U.S. Government Printing Office, 1982.

Department of the Army. *Leaders' Manual for Combat Stress Control*. FM 22-51. Washington, D.C.: U.S. Government Printing Office, 1994.

Department of the Army. *Medical Platoon Leaders' Handbook*. FM 4-02.4. Washington, D.C.: U.S. Government Printing Office, 2001.

Department of the Army. *Prevention and Management of Cold-Weather Injuries*. TB MED 508. Washington, D.C.: U.S. Government Printing Office, 2005.

Department of the Army. *US Army Survival Manual*. FM 21-76. Washington, D.C.: U.S. Government Printing Office, 1970.

Department of the Army. *Unit Field Sanitation Teams*. ATP 4-25.12. Washington, D.C.: U.S. Government Printing Office, 2014.

Department of the Army and Air Force. *Heat Stress Control and Heat Casualty Management*. TB MED 507/AFPAM 48-152 (I). Washington, D.C.: U.S. Government Printing Office, 2003.

Department of the Army and the Marine Corps. FM 90-3/FMFM 7-27. Washington, D.C.: U.S. Government Printing Office, 1993.

Department of the Army, Marine Corps Combat Development Command, Department of the Navy, and U.S. Marine Corps. *Cold Region Operations*. ATTP 3-97.11/MCRP 3-35.1D. Washington, D.C.: U.S. Government Printing Office, 2011.

Departments of the Army, the Navy, and the Air Force. *First Aid*. FM 4-25.11/ NTRP 4-02.1/AFMAN 44-163(I). Washington, D.C.: U.S. Government Printing Office, 2002.

Pipeline and Hazardous Materials Safety Administration, U.S. Department of Transportation. *2016 Emergency Response Guidebook*. ERG2016. Washington, D.C.: U.S. Government Printing Office, 2016.

Special Operations Command, Department of Defense. *Special Operations Forces Medical Handbook*. Washington, D.C.: U.S. Government Printing Office, 2001.

U.S. Marine Corps. *Summer Survival Course Handbook*. MSVX.02.01. Bridgeport, CA: Mountain Warfare Training Center, 2005.

OTHER RESOURCES

Brown, Tom. *Tom Brown's Guide to Wild Edible and Medicinal Plants*. New York: Berkley, 1985.

Foster, Steven, and James A. Duke. *Peterson Field Guide to Medicinal Plants and Herbs of Eastern and Central North America*. 3rd ed. New York: Houghton Mifflin Harcourt, 2014.

Kragh, John F. Jr., Thomas J. Walters, David G. Baer, Charles E. Wade, Jose Salinas, and John B. Holcomb. "Survival with emergency tourniquet use to stop bleeding in major limb trauma." *Annals of Surgery* 249, no. 1 (Jan 2009): 1-7.

McCullough, Jay, ed. *The Ultimate Guide to U.S. Army Survival Skills, Tactics, and Techniques*. New York: Skyhorse Publishing, 2007.

Tawrell, Paul. *Camping & Wilderness Survival*. 2nd ed. Shelburne, VT: Paul Tawrell, 2006.

Thayer, Samuel. *The Forager's Harvest: A Guide to Identifying, Harvesting, and Preparing Edible Wild Plants*. Ogema, WI: Forager's Harvest, 2006.

Triservice Nursing Research Program. *Battlefield and Disaster Nursing Pocket Guide*. Sudbury, MA: Jones and Bartlett Publishers, 2009.

Williams, Scott B. and Scott Finazzo. *The Prepper's Workbook*. Berkeley, CA: Ulysses Press, 2014.

Wiseman, John "Lofty." *SAS Survival Handbook: The Ultimate Guide to Surviving Anywhere*. 3rd ed. New York: William Morrow Paperbacks, 2014.

INDEX

Note: In general, specific field manuals used as sources are not indexed here.

ACKNOWLEDGMENTS

First and foremost, I would like to thank all at Ulysses Press for their vision and trust in me to write this book. Special thanks to Caety Klingman for her patience and hard work to make this project what it has become. Additional thanks to all who have contributed or supported me throughout this process: my family, my sons Ryan, Nicholas, and Cameron, my OPFD family, Angela Caruso-Yahne, Randy Pommenville, Scott B. Williams, and Julie Harper.

ABOUT THE AUTHOR

Scott Finazzo has been a firefighter for nearly 20 years and is currently serving as a lieutenant for the Overland Park, Kansas, Fire Department. He has been an instructor for firefighting tactics, confined space rescue, first aid, CPR, Community Emergency Response Teams, and other emergency training. In addition to being an emergency responder and educator, Scott has been writing in various capacities for much of his life, contributing to blogs, magazines, and books. Scott's first book, co-authored with Scott B. Williams, *The Prepper's Workbook*, became a national best seller. He followed that up with the narrative of his kayak journey through the Virgin Islands called *Why Do All the Locals Think We're Crazy?* Most recently he wrote *The Neighborhood Emergency Response Handbook* and he is currently writing the manuscript for his upcoming book *Prepper's Guide to Knots*.

Scott has a bachelor's degree in management and human relations, and two associate degrees. Follow him at www.scottfinazzo.com.

CPSIA information can be obtained
at www.ICGtesting.com
Printed in the USA
LVHW031010231121
704194LV00002B/6

9 781612 435657